THE LITTLE BOOK OF NITS

Look... Find... Remove... Rejoice...
Eat only if really necessary

RICHARD JONES AND JUSTINE CROW

BLOOMSBURY
LONDON · BERLIN · NEW YORK · SYDNEY.

First published in Great Britain 2012 by
Bloomsbury Publishing Plc
50 Bedford Square
London WC1B 3DP
www.bloomsbury.com

Copyright © 2012 Richard Jones
and Justine Crow

ISBN 978-1-4081-5550-9

The authors have asserted their rights
under the Copyright, Design and
Patents Act, 1988, to be identified as
the authors of this work.

Commissioning editor: Jim Martin
Page design: Susan McIntyre
Project editor: Jasmine Parker

Printed and bound in Great Britain by
Clays Limited, St Ives plc

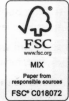

FSC
www.fsc.org
MIX
Paper from
responsible sources
FSC® C018072

Contents

Before we get down to business...

With thanks to all my friends who have provided me with an endless supply of nitty anecdotes over the years, provoking much snotty laughter over a glass or two. And thanks also to those who gave me help in those early dark days of infestation.

Strangely, I also give thanks to the lice for forcing me – yes, forcing me – to spend some kind of quality time with my kids while we combed. No, really. We talked, we bathed, we joked, we gasped in awe. We wept at the end of *The Railway Children* every time we watched it while slathered in conditioner. We giggled at the secret scratch that happened in places where people weren't supposed to know we had a head full, and we luxuriated in joint relief when a comb-through refused to yield a single bug. Until the next time

Justine Crow

On 13 March 1986, I had arranged for Professor John Maunder of Cambridge University to give a lecture to the British Entomological and Natural History Society in the elegant hall of the Alpine Club in London's West End. Unfortunately, several inches of snow fell on London that day and there were only five of us in the audience. Nevertheless, Professor Maunder put on his best show. That lecture – and his similarly-titled article on 'The Appreciation of Lice', published in the *Proceedings of the Royal Institution* – have long been a personal inspiration to me. I'm afraid I've used it for more than its fair share of facts and figures here. So I salute his wit, knowledge and experience and offer this small book as flattery of his work.

Richard Jones ➤ *Bugman*

DON'T PANIC!

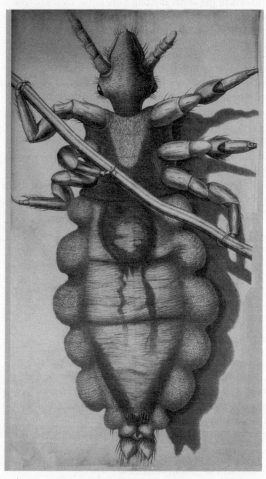

It's not a monster...

Oh dear. One of the children has come home from school with the usual head louse letter. It may be helpful and suggest all manner of preparations and treatments to get rid of the blighters. Or it might accuse you of being a *bad parent* and endangering the health, safety and good name of the school. Whatever. DON'T PANIC!

Much of what you know, or think you know, about head lice is going to be wrong. There are so many quack cures and old wives' tales that sorting fact from fiction is sometimes very difficult.

But congratulations, you have taken the right first step in picking up this little book. It's time to start getting our facts straight.

First, head lice are very common. They are *particularly* common amongst schoolchildren. Rough estimates suggest that almost 40% of children will get head lice at some point between the ages of three and ten.

Second, they are easy to catch ⇒ almost as easy as catching a cold. Anyone from presidents to paupers can catch a cold, and they can get head lice, too.

Third, head lice are not choosy about whose head they infest. From baker to barrister, we can all get head lice; even entomologists get head lice.

Lastly, they can be got rid of.

We take care not to peddle any particular product with this book. And we distance ourselves from anyone else promoting particular potions, poisons or gadgets. But there is only one sure-fire way of ridding yourselves and your families of head lice. That is to understand what these tiny critters are, how they live, how they breed and how they move about.

Then you can set about removing them.

Don't *Get*
Muddled

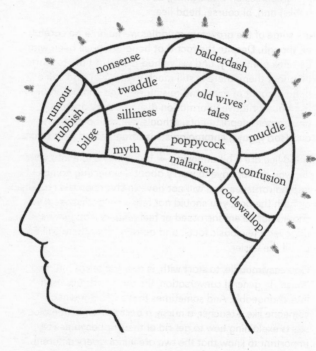

James, (aged six) on his way home from school: Mum, I had a letter from the teacher to give you, but I lost it.

Edwina: Oh! What did it say?

James: It said you have to look in my hair for woodlice.

James can be forgiven his childish muddle. 'Louse' is an old word and it's used for all sorts of small, mean, crawling creatures. Apart from woodlice – the familiar, domed crustaceans living under logs in the garden – there are hoglice (water woodlice), fish-lice (flat prawn-like fish parasites), plant-lice (a bit like greenflies), bark-lice (a bit like greenflies on tree trunks), booklice (inhabitants of old books) and, of course, head lice.

It's some of the grown-up muddles we have to be careful of, though. Despite the fact that head lice have been with us since prehistory, and we've had plenty of time to learn all about them, there is still much to discover and still a huge amount of myth and misinformation spread around. Even authoritative information dished out by doctors, government departments, schools, education authorities and (sorry, guys) entomologists is often littered with errors.

Head lice are a bit annoying ➡ but if they come into your life, you do not have to worry about disinfecting combs and hairbrushes; you will not have to shampoo the carpets or bath the dog; you should not feel dirty or diseased; you should not be embarrassed or feel unlucky. You just need to discover a few basic facts, and getting rid of them will then be all the easier.

One easy muddle, to start with, is over the terms 'nit' and 'louse'. In general conversation, the two words are used interchangeably. And sometimes that's OK. But when someone like a teacher, a nurse, a doctor or an entomologist starts explaining how to get rid of them, it becomes very important to know that the two are, in fact, very different. And neither is anything to do with woodlice.

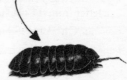

WHAT IS A NIT?

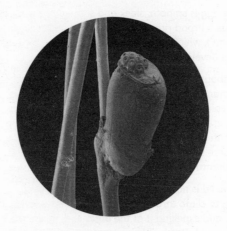

What came first?
The louse or the nit?

A nit is a louse egg. More particularly, it is an *empty* louse egg-shell, because by the time the nit is spotted, the tiny louseling has hatched out and crawled off across the scalp. Strictly speaking, an egg with a louse embryo still inside does not have its own name, but let's not split hairs over this (or the nits attached to them).

A nit is tiny. At 0.8 by 0.3mm, it's about the size of the full stop at the end of this sentence. To put a nit in perspective, a hen's egg is over one and a half million times the size, a goose egg is four million times as big and an ostrich egg – should you have one lying about in the kitchen – is 43 million times the size of a nit.

The louse egg is smooth, sleek and shaped like a rugby ball. It has a broad rimmed neck and a flip-top lid (the 'operculum'), which has about 16 small holes, through which the developing louse embryo breathes.

It takes about a week from egg laying to louse hatching. The optimum temperature for development is 31°C, which is coincidentally very similar to the usual scalp temperature of 33°C. Louse eggs do not hatch below 22°C. Unfortunately, unless you sleep with your head in the fridge, there is no way you can get your scalp down to this temperature.

Oddly, the lid is not quite big enough for the louse hatchling to climb through. Instead, it starts swallowing down air and expelling it at the other end, inside the base of the eggshell. This builds up pressure inside the nit, enough to push out the louse like a cork from a champagne bottle.

There is no pop and no airborne trajectory, but what a neat trick.

WHAT IS A HEAD LOUSE?

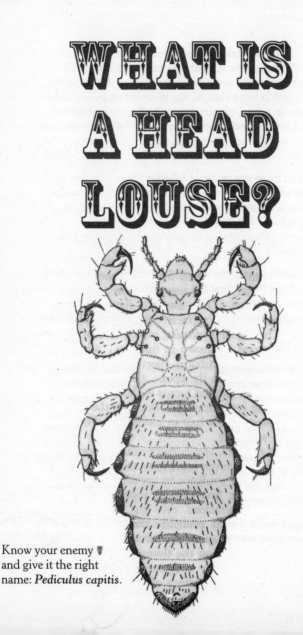

Know your enemy
and give it the right
name: *Pediculus capitis*.

The human head louse *Pediculus capitis* is a tiny (3.3mm at the biggest), narrow, wingless, blood-sucking insect with short antennae and stout legs, each ending with a large claw. In life, the head louse is a dull pale cream colour, perfectly described in one Victorian monograph as 'cadaverous ashy white'. Its body is actually opaque and the narrow dark squiggle seen in its abdomen is its gut, with the remnants of your blood being digested.

The head louse is a rather soft-bodied insect. Its skin is flexible and elastic, unlike the tough armoured carapace of those other bloodsuckers, the flea or the bedbug. It does, however, have some very tough parts of its body – its gripping claws and its sucking mouthparts, more on them later.

Head lice belong to the insect order Phthiraptera, a name coined from the Ancient Greek word for louse, *phtheir*. When said with a slight lisp and a nasal sneer, it makes just the right sound for such a revolting parasite – phtheir. It also gives us the job title 'phthirapterist' ← someone who studies lice.

There have been arguments over head lice for as long as there have been phthirapterists. The problem is that the human head louse looks extremely similar to the human *body* louse, *Pediculus humanus* (see pages 102–7), even under a powerful microscope. In the laboratory, head and body lice will interbreed to give intermediate lice. In the past, head lice were sometimes thought to be a subspecies, or race, of body lice and called *Pediculus humanus* form *capitis*, while the body-inhabiting insects were P*ediculus humanus* form *corporis*.

But don't worry. If you find lice on a head, they are head lice. It's simple.

HAVE WE GOT NITS?

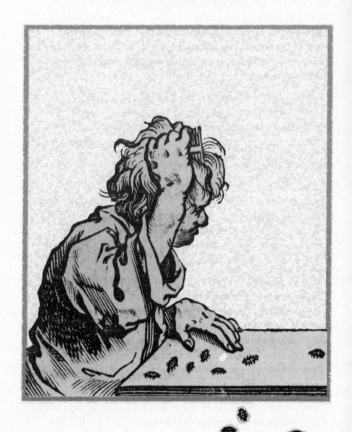

Scratching is not the first sign of infestation but it is often the first noticeable symptom. Unfortunately, by the time the host starts feeling the itch, the head lice have usually got a very good toe-hold.

Nits are very difficult to see. The empty shells where lice have hatched look white or cream coloured on the shaft of the hair; the live nits yet to emerge are darker. The louse lays eggs close to the scalp, so often the nit isn't obvious until the hair has grown away from the head. By then, several generations of lice may have laid and hatched and lots of empty nit shells are visible, looking like salt grains glued to the hair.

Check behind the ears, the nape of the neck and the parting of the hair; these are favoured, though by no means exclusive, haunts of the louse.

Spotting a live insect is also difficult unless the host has an acute infestation. Do not rely on your eyesight or Holmesian skills of deduction.

The best way to identify infestation is by wet combing after applying a slippery base (like conditioner) and then wiping the comb after each stroke on a tissue or cloth. The live insects vary in size – the fully developed adult is about the same size as a fennel seed, or a cat flea, and pale reddish-brown with visible legs.

Freshly-hatched lice are absolutely tiny and, in their way, as cute as kittens. On tissue, they will appear as black specks, smaller than pepper grounds. Eggs are less easily combed out (that special louse glue is tenacious stuff, see page 20) but with perseverance, they can be removed. Sometimes a live egg will make a satisfying popping sound when cracked between the backs of your thumbnails.

If you discover that nits and/or lice are present, deal with the problem as soon possible because otherwise the lice will continue to multiply and spread...

Lousiness is Next to Cleanliness

'In some societies, the act of grooming for nits is deemed a perfectly acceptable social activity and why not? One Asian mother I spoke to at nursery said she had happy memories of cracking the nits in her dad's hair. Another mother said she derives immense pleasure from sliding the live nits off her children's hair with her nail tips and then trying to elicit the "little snap" from each one.'

Theresa, Croydon

'On occasion, I have been asked to check my friends' heads over a glass of wine in the kitchen. It is a necessity and we always have a laugh about it. After all, if you have kids you are going to catch nits at some time or another, but how can you check the back of your own head?'

Helen, Croydon

A piece of advice if your children are about to begin primary school ➡ make sure you always have a nit comb and tissues. But no matter how prepared you are, the first time your child gets nits is always a surprise. If it happens, remember that you are not a bad parent. Infestation is an inevitable part of growing up. If we arm ourselves with the facts, then we can deal with the problem once we get over the shock of it.

NIT MYTH
Head Lice Are Dirty

🕯 Head lice like heads. Whether they are clean or dirty heads – lice don't have a preference. While it is true they flourish in the warm, moist conditions on the scalp, they also require pretty precise temperature and humidity to survive. You can make life nigh on impossible for lice to proliferate by the simple act of combing with a fine-toothed comb once a week.

🕯 Nits and lice cannot be 'washed off' with water, nor can they be drowned. Occasionally a live louse may get brushed out, but you can keep your hair as clean and tidy as you like and it will not keep the critters away. Washing your hair once a day or once a year makes no difference.

🕯 The current resurgence we appear to be experiencing has everything to do with our notions of our own hygiene – 'it can't happen to us!' – and our expectations of the efficacy of over-the-counter products once infestation does occur. While there is *some* reliable historical data showing that head lice infestation was once more common among the poor because they were forced to share beds and live in squalid conditions, there is also most definitely a case for arguing that once upon a time families were more skilled at recognising symptoms and treating them because they had no recourse to a pharmacist or doctor.

🕯 Our reluctance to use routine grooming as a preventative measure – despite our desire to rid ourselves of unclean beasts – is evident in the amount we spend in the chemist on anti-louse shampoos in the hope of an instant cure.

🕯 It makes sense to keep haircuts short, manageable and tangle-free – especially in school-age children – so that when infestation occurs, you are not tearing out your hair (or indeed theirs) in your attempts to deal with it.

The *Perfect* Glue

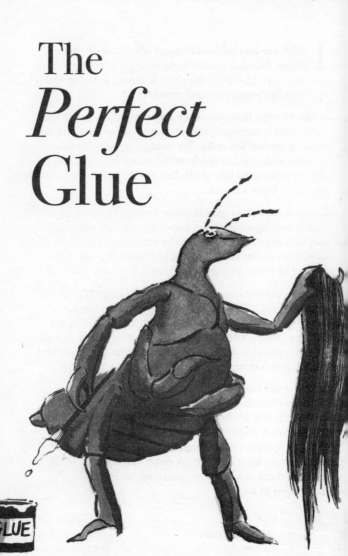

Lice are very particular about where they lay their eggs. An adult female louse lays just a few eggs (perhaps only 55–60 in her short lifetime), but each one is laid with deliberate care and attention.

A human head louse lays each egg somewhere warm and moist. This is usually right at the very base of a human hair, hard up against the scalp. The loving mother louse sticks it in place with a tough, quick-setting glue that forms a tight sheath around the hair shaft. This special glue is one of the secrets of louse success.

The glue is made in glands inside the louse's abdomen. Like that other important insect secretion, silk, it is squeezed out as a liquid, but quickly hardens on contact with air. The female louse has two special appendages ('gonopods') on her tail to smear and wrap the glue around the hair stalk.

This egg cement has spawned plenty of research projects. Technically, it is 'composed of four bands of protein, possibly cross-linked to aliphatic components with a tertiary structure of beta sheeting'. In other words, it is a highly complex compound, and very similar in its chemical make-up to human hair.

This is good news for the louse, because it means that the glue attaching the egg grips extremely tightly to the hair stand. It's bad news for the pharmaceutical companies trying to develop nit-removing shampoos, though. It means that chemicals likely to break down the cement *also* attack and break down human hair. So far, none of these supposed nit-loosening lotions show any such signs of success.

LOUSE LIFE

The Life of a Louse

A drama in three acts

ACT I The Hair of the Head – A Simple Place But Warm and Cosy

The Nit A louse egg

The Nymph A baby louse

The Head Louse The villain (*audience boos and hisses*)

ACT II The Infestation – It's Getting Mighty Crowded

The Head Lice   Lots of them, feasting and fornicating

The Nymphs   They're everywhere

The Nits   Too many to count

ACT III The Denouement

Enter:

The Nit Comb The hero (*audience cheers and applauds*)

Cue: dramatic sweeping music

Lice, nymphs and nits exit stage left, pursued by comb

Head lice spend a lot of time having sex. Female insects usually have a sperm-storage organ (spermathaeca), and one mating is often enough to fertilise all the eggs they will lay in their entire lives. But in head lice, the part of the reproductive tract that ought to be a spermathaeca is so small its existence was long denied by louse researchers. One or two fertile eggs are laid after each mating; rarely three, never four. Anyway, they spend a lot of time at it. To save time, they usually feed while mating.

Eggs (nits) are laid at a rate of about 6–10 a day, mostly at night. The eggs start to hatch in around seven to nine days. Lice do not go through a magical metamorphosis like caterpillar to butterfly; instead, the baby louseling, the nymph, is already a miniature version of the adult. It starts feeding immediately. The newly hatched lice are about 1mm long ← roughly the size of the commas on this page. They are a devil of a job to spot.

After two days (about 10 blood meals), the louse nymph outgrows its skin, which splits open and is cast off. It will shed its skin twice more before reaching adulthood; the whole process takes about 10 days.

The empty skins discarded by the moulting lice are whisper-thin but they retain the size and exact shape of the louse down to the last claw, like a louse 'ghost'. In very heavy infestations, these empty skins can be seen on our shoulders or pillows. It is these which probably gave rise to the myths about 'wind-blown transfer' or contamination via hats and hair-bands.

One generation of head lice takes just two or three weeks to change from newly deposited nit to sexually hyperactive adult＊

DON'T FUSS OVER EMPTY EGGSHELLS

DID YOU KNOW?

Aristotle had nits. Or his children did. Or his pupils, maybe.

Anyway, he knew they were produced by head lice, but he wasn't quite sure exactly what they were.

He thought that head lice appeared, spontaneously, from the scalp (something to do with the reaction of the skin and the moisture within).

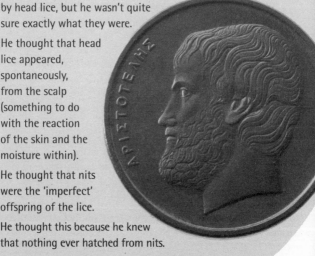

He thought that nits were the 'imperfect' offspring of the lice.

He thought this because he knew that nothing ever hatched from nits.

That's because they had *already* hatched DUMBO▾

Nits are empty eggshells. It's the *live* head lice you need to look for. The trouble is that nits are very obvious, and lice are not. When the eggs were laid, they were a dull grey, and they blended in perfectly against the scalp. Now they are empty, bright white and stand out like beacons.

Nits can remain attached to hair strands for months. We have that excellent nit glue to thank for that, and there they remain – as obvious as ever, until we do something about it.

As the hair grows, the nits move further away from the scalp. Human hair grows about 13mm per month. So four months after they were laid, the nits will be about 50mm along the hair. This also gives the impression that head lice live up in the thick hair. But head lice live on the scalp; this is the place, after all, from which the blood is sucked.

Nits' brilliant whiteness is no accident. While the lice can hide safely, scurrying about on the scalp and hidden under the hair thatch, the nits now become the perfect target for any grooming. They are so easy to see that they divert attention away from the lice at play beneath them.

But, they can also linger on ➤ long after the lice that laid them have been combed away. It suddenly becomes clear that a 'no nits' policy in schools is pointless. Nits are empty eggshells. They are left over even after the head lice may have been removed. The living head lice are the things that bite, that itch and that move about from head to head.

Look for *living* lice ➤

Head
Banging

NIT MYTH

Girls Get Nits More Often Than Boys

It is claimed that girls suffer head lice more frequently that boys. This is perfectly possible, but not because their hair is any more enticing to a head louse. Pretty or long hair makes no difference to infestation levels – it is more likely because girls' social behaviour is more tactile than boys.

Then there is the much dreaded (by parents) cultural phenomenon of THE SLEEPOVER. Once, one only stayed at a friend's house when there was an emergency, such as an imminent birth or an unexpected death. A bed was usually made up modestly on the floor or downstairs on a couch. Not today, as you will have experienced (or will do soon). These days the sleepover is one of childhood's exquisite experiences. Several children at a time crowd under a single duvet in front of a DVD; tents in back gardens are filled with airbeds ready to burst under the combined weight of excited campers; living room floors are criss-crossed with sleeping bags. Oh, those lucky old head lice love a sleepover.

These days, there are seemingly many more opportunities for heads to come together. Head lice love the new learning curriculum. Gone are the days when each child sat separately at school in silence and faced the stark blackboard at individual flip-up wooden desks. Modern learning happens in small huddles around tables where head-to-head contact is inevitable. Mentoring is a system currently favoured in primary and secondary schools where pupils are encouraged to work together over books and at computer screens. There are group discussions and plenty of talking. Teachers get nits too, all the time. Ask one about it.

Ah. Computer screens. And consoles. It is very common these days for children to play electronic games together, side-by-side on a sofa, flopping around and having fun with plenty of contact. Once, this kind of familiarity was frowned upon. Now, leisure activities of this type are utterly normal.

Boys have traditionally enjoyed more 'rough and tumble' than their female counterparts. But while this used to be confined to the playground and back gardens, in today's age of controlled exercise and myriad after-school activities – art clubs, computer clubs, homework clubs, breakfast clubs and so on – there are scores of daily opportunities for boys' and girls' heads to come together. And of course, nature will step in to take advantage.

There is also a theory that our wider family represents a constant supply of head lice. It is believed (by some) that grandparents and other older relatives possibly harbour 'benign colonies' of lice whose numbers remain low on the host's head, but then rapidly spread to the grandchildren where their numbers increase. I am sorry to say that the term 'benign colonies' has entered into the Crow household vernacular whenever the subject of granddad or grandma is raised.

HOW DO LICE SPREAD?

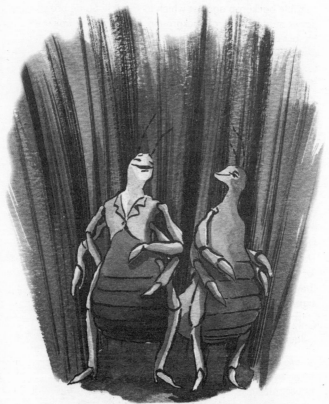

"So, do you come here often?"

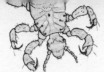

Lice crawl. They are very good at it. One look at the giant claws at the end of their legs shows that these formidable grappling irons could be used for nothing except gripping very tightly. Head lice are, nevertheless, very nimble.

When I wanted to photograph a live head louse plucked from one of my children's heads, I looked about for a suitable backdrop against which to shoot it. Some brown paper made a neutral background, but the louse was a bit lost against the flat expanse of buff. Ah, but then I remembered the clippings from the kids' recent haircuts, tossed into the garden. I gathered up a sprig of hairs, scattered them on the paper and released the louse.

It rushed off immediately across the jumbled strands surprisingly fast as I tried to get it in focus for a portrait. Each time it got to the end of a hair, it stopped and tore off in the other direction. It kept swapping from one hair to another; up, down, left, right. I took the pictures I needed. The louse kept going. It did not stop but neither did it ever let go of a hair and walk off across the paper. For 20 minutes it continued its frantic exploration of the cut strands. Never did it relinquish its grip.

Head lice do not waltz across the pillow or the chair back. They wait until there is the opportunity to crawl. They wait for the necessary head-to-head contact. They wait until they can grip the hair strand of the new victim. Then they scramble across very nimbly.

Only death – either their own or their host's – will ever induce a head louse to let go.

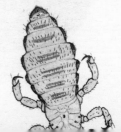

LETTING GO IS SUICIDE

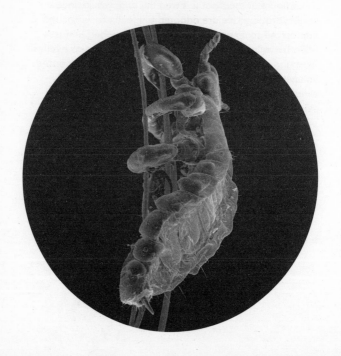

A louse is a tiny parasite in a giant world. A head louse does not decide to go walking off the head to lie in wait on pieces of furniture until another head comes along. Head lice are small, soft and vulnerable. They would just get squashed if they tried it, or they would get lost.

A human is about 100 million times the size of a head louse. That's roughly the same size differential as that between a human and a cruise liner. No person in their right mind would dive off a liner in the middle of the ocean in the hope of being picked up by another one swinging past later. It would be suicide.

Just as the human could not survive very long in the sea, a louse cannot survive very long away from the head — a few hours at the most if it were lucky. It would soon die of dehydration. Lice are adapted to life in the warm, moist hair on the scalp and there is always liquid refreshment (blood) available. Unlike free-living insects such as beetles, bees and butterflies, the soft-bodied louse cannot control its own water loss – it does not need to. Away from the climate-controlled comfort of the human head, it would soon dry out.

It would get cold, too. The human scalp is a more or less constant 33°C. The back of a chair is 10°C lower, even on a warm day. The louse's metabolic processes would become corrupted and slowed, as would its body movements. It very soon grinds to a halt.

The hair on the scalp is safe. Letting go would be suicide.

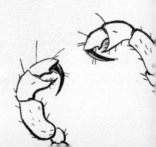

ARE WE BAD PARENTS?

NIT MYTH

Blonde Children Don't Get Nits

All children can get nits, regardless of complexion, ethnic background, creed or religion. We live in an increasingly urban environment with sterile and relentlessly disinfected homes. Finding insects indoors is bad enough. Finding them on our children's heads is really disturbing. It doesn't help that they are so hard to see until it is too late. For something so elusive, they sure have presence.

The earliest known relationship between the humble head louse and a human being was discovered when the remains of a nit attached to a human hair were found at an archaeological dig in South America. The nit was thought to be 10,000 years old.

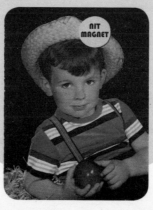

From our blog

When was your first time?

My friend Alice said her first time was 10 years ago when her eldest daughter, then aged six, came home from school with the standard generic note about a reported case of infestation. She gave her little head the once over, spotted nothing and forgot all about it. Two weeks later, she said there were head lice practically abseiling off her daughter's eyebrows. She said she felt terrible. The kid was teeming – it was a veritable louse circus with insects swinging off her hair like they were on a trapeze. Why hadn't she noticed them before?

I have an image of my youngest sister in my head, unkempt as a feral kitten, mute til she was five (she couldn't get a word in edgewise with four older siblings and umpteen adults all over the house), with a stinking chemical potion simmering on her head. I remember thinking, ha ha. I'm so glad that's not me, until my mother beckoned me into the bathroom to take a turn.

In those days, there were no niceties with a nit comb. If you got that brown envelope from school, it meant the nit nurse had spoken and my mum – squeamish about creepy crawlies at the best of times – applied the regulation sheep dip without hesitation. And that stuff reeked so much it howled. What did they put in it? Napalm?

It was treatment of the herd, regardless of whether there were any signs of life in any other familial thatch and it was the same when she came home with worms. I can still taste the warm blackcurrant mix in the paper cup we all had to gag down. To this day I can't smell – let alone drink – Ribena without wanting to retch. Vile...

We are not bad parents if our children get nits. We are bad parents if we share our vodka and fags with them.

Teasing, Bullying and Social Stigma

WHAT TO DO?

The stigmatisation of head lice comes from adults, not children. Any teasing – or worse, bullying – by children about someone having nits is caused by the disgust reflex of the adults around them.

❀ If you discover your child has a head full, try not to gag in front of them. In general, having nits doesn't bother children in the slightest but it drives mums and dads to distraction.

❀ Be honest, as honest as you can bear. Warn fellow parents and carers that you have discovered lice or nits in your child's hair and that everybody needs to be treated.

❀ Offer to help others coping with an infestation. Long-sighted people dread nits because they can't see them. Others are squeamish. Yet more are ill-informed.

❀ Mass combing is fun. No kidding, it can be a social occasion. Get the kids round the table and get several adults combing. Who has got the most?

❀ Official bug combing days are a great way of reducing the stigma. A school signs up and each pupil comes home with a comb, a leaflet and a prescribed date for everyone to adhere to.

❀ Don't be ashamed. Cavemen had nits, as did aristocrats in the Renaissance. Think how many celebrities have had their mums or babysitters groan at the sight of a little hand going up behind the ear for a good scratch.

'My daughter Lucy hadn't yet contracted head lice, so I was a bit surprised when a friend mentioned to me that Lucy had told her little girl Ellie that she also had nits, imagining that perhaps one had passed them to the other. When I asked Lucy why she had told Ellie's mum this, she looked baffled. "Because I have," she replied and tugged at her long, blonde curly hair, "and they get all tangled". I then realised what she meant. "You had knots!" I laughed. "Yes, that's what I said. Knots." But the truth is, nits or knots, Lucy was just happy to be the same as Ellie.'

Connie, Dulwich

'I was a designated parent on a school trip to a museum and as there were odd numbers, I sat next to a neighbour's little girl while my son bounced around at the back of the coach with his friend. As the journey progressed, I watched in horrified fascination as big, fat head lice began patrolling her middle parting. I didn't say anything to her about this at the time but once the trip was over, I took a deep breath and rang their doorbell. Well, if it was my child, I'd want to know…'

Janice, Beckenham

'The kids had head lice at home and one brave day, we decided to examine one under the microscope my eldest had got for Christmas. There it was, unbelievably huge and magnified on a strand of hair. We watched it scuttle up and down athletically. Then I moved backwards slightly and the hair shifted under the lens and I realised it was my hair it was doing tricks on. Somehow, in leaning in closely, I had offered it the ideal passage from head to head.'

Judith, Dulwich

'I like my nits, they are like pets you can give to other people.'
Alice, 7¼ years old

WHEN

DADDY

GOT NITS

NIT MYTH ❦ TRUE OR FALSE?

Men Don't Get Nits Because of Their Hormones

False: This is pernicious rubbish. Basically blokes, especially dads, get nits less often because they do not put their heads next to their kids' heads as regularly as mums, aunties and nans do. Liking football and pot noodles is no protection.

From our blog

The key to keeping on top of nits is preparation. Thus, my bathroom cupboard always contains a selection of trusty combs, cheap tissues and, most importantly, a bargain conditioner. I find the bottom end of the supermarket range is the slimiest and you can slather it on without feeling remorseful about the price. Thus equipped, you are instantly armed to respond at the first sign of attack.

On one occasion, my partner Jon announced that as everyone else had been raked, it was his turn. But rather than let the queen of the comb (me) near his bald patch, he was going to do his own head. So, I left him running the taps.

A quarter of an hour later there was a hefty groan from the bathroom, followed by 'Juuusssttiinne!' Naturally, I came running, followed by three curious children, and we entered the steamy bathroom to find Daddy in the bath, staring at a piece of wilting tissue. We all looked. The tissue was smeared with hundreds of tiny black bits. The children were incredibly impressed, saying 'wowser!' and 'corrr!' and eventually they struck up a chirpy chorus of 'Daddy's got nits, Daddy's got nits'.

I shooed the kids away and took the tissue for a closer look. 'Er, darling? Which conditioner did you use?' I asked, surveying the array of bargain gunk and posh unguents.

'The Body Shop banana one,' he replied glumly, preparing the comb for another sweep.

'Banana?' I laughed. 'That'll be the one full of little black seeds, then.'

'Yes,' he confirmed, miserably pulling another cheap tissue from the box. I quietly shut the door and waited on the landing while the penny dropped▾

> *'I suspect that most entomologists
> have never seen a head louse –
> perhaps this is because they
> are mostly men.'*

NITS IN THE CLASSROOM

There is misinformation and perpetuation of the myths concerning lice infestation everywhere, including the one place where accurate education really matters ➤ school.

This whimsical suggestion was sent out to every child in one Southwark primary school:

Headmaster's Nit Homework

25 drops rosemary oil

25 drops lavender oil

13 drops geranium oil

12 drops eucalyptus oil

75 ml almond oil

Mix oils together. Soak hair with the mixture, cover hair with cling film then shampoo out. Repeat three days later.

If nothing else, the pong will knock 'em out.

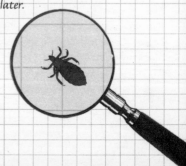

'I actually heard an adult – a nursery nurse, in fact – tell a parent that she didn't ever get nits because she had blonde hair. I was shocked that the woman was peddling such twaddle. It's not surprising the pre-school had so many cases of head lice.'

Mike, Nottingham

'When my boy got nits, I spent the evening combing as they say you should and when he went to school the next morning, I had a discreet word with his teacher. According to school policy, parents are supposed to inform the teacher when their child gets head lice so that he or she can give out the school advice letter at the end of the day. When my son got home with the requisite note about what action to take, I asked him what, if anything, his teacher had said to him. "She didn't say anything to me," he replied, "but when she took the register, she asked all the children in the class who had nits to put their hands up." "And did anyone else put their hand up apart from you?" I enquired. "Oh yes," he answered solemnly. "About 12 did."'

Lynne, Reigate

'My son came home from school saying, "Mum, I've got nits". I said, "don't be silly. How could you have them?" You see, he isn't the most sociable child; he's fairly shy and rarely has friends over for tea. He said, "I was doing maths and scratched my head and one fell onto my page. It was brilliant!"'

Katherine, Horsham

Keeping Warm and Moist

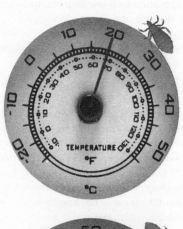

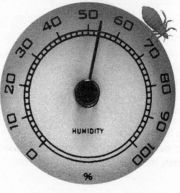

Head lice have got it made. They live in the perfect habitat, maintained like a climate-controlled apartment, at exactly the right temperature and comfortable humidity, and food is on tap all day long. But this life of luxury has made lice negligent in their survival mechanisms. Change their environment, even a little bit, and they are in big trouble.

Drop the temperature by a few degrees, for example, and they become sluggish and clumsy. Mating stops, fertility drops and eggs start failing. Raise it and the lice start panicking: they flee from dangerously feverish heads like rats leaving a sinking ship.

Humidity is their greatest worry, though. Lice live on a liquid diet, but their nice, comfortable home would soon become mired with slimy goo if they passed copious sticky faeces. Instead, they lose most of the water from their blood meals by evaporating it directly out through their soft, porous skin, which means they can pass dry, dusty pellets that do not clog their home or stick to their feet. This was the 'nitty-gritty' disturbed by the heavily louse-infested schoolchild scratching his or her head when struggling over reading, 'riting and 'rithmetic.

But remove a louse from its warm moist scalp, with its plentiful supply of liquid food, and this same evaporation mechanism places it in immediate danger of drying out. A head louse removed from a head will be dead within 24–36 hours, but desiccation sets in much faster – within three to five hours, in fact – and lice become unable to feed because of dehydration long before they stop moving.

The writhing legs of a head louse caught on the tines of a comb are its last frantic dying struggles. A louse removed from its homely head of hair is doomed✶

Hairbrushes, Hats and *Antimacassars*

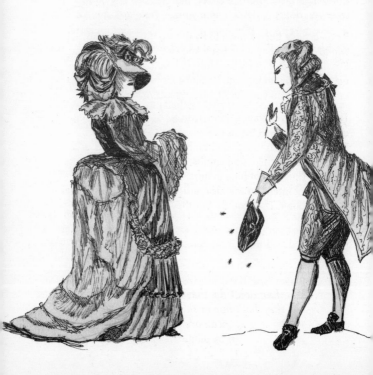

A **question** often repeated by hard-pressed parents and carers runs something along the following lines: can my child catch head lice from cuddly toys/ hats/ scarves/ pillows/ blankets/ chairs/ school desks/ in fact almost anything? Time and again, studies show that lice spreading on these objects is as rare as hen's teeth.

Unfortunately, even books by experts usually say something like 'louse transmission can occur via shared objects such as combs, brushes, headphones and hats'. Note the 'can'. They *can*, but they don't. Not really.

How would it look if, sitting in my kitchen writing this book, I have an umbrella up to protect me against pigeon droppings? I could argue that a pigeon might fly in through the open doors and poop on my head. It *could* happen.

Pigeons have been known to fly in through doors and windows. And they have been known to poop on heads. But if I were to write a book about kitchens and warn that umbrellas should be used because birds can sometimes fly in and dump on your head, I would look a right twit.

There are lots of things head lice can do, but don't. They do not dance. They do not move south for the winter. They do not go hang-gliding on hairs cut at the barber's. They do not hitch lifts on combs, hairbrushes or headphones. They do not hide in hats. They do not loiter with malevolent intent on the lacy antimacassar on the back of the easy chair. They could. But they don't.

> 'Lice don't fly, they don't jump,
> they don't hop or skip or vault –
> they sneak around as
> if by magic.'

SHAVING CAN HELP

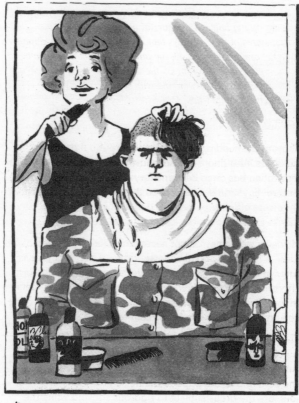

"Going anywhere nice on your Tour of Duty?"

'I know somebody who has been thrown out of every hairdresser in town for having head lice. Even though I can't imagine anything more embarrassing, she just laughs it off. It still doesn't shame her into treating her own head, let alone her children's.'

Anna, Dulwich

'My friend Dee is a stylist at a salon, but she makes a good living cutting hair out of hours in people's homes because she isn't scared of nits. She says that as long as she makes certain all her combs are rinsed off, she can't see the problem and other hairdressers are ignorant of the facts. And she's brilliant at chasing small children around with scissors! I don't know how she gets a straight fringe…'

Dawn, Wandsworth

Shaving the head is an effective – if brutal – way of getting rid of lice infestation. Indeed, shaving new recruits to prevent infestation has often been military policy. It is thought that Ancient Egyptian priests shaved their heads completely if they were afflicted by nymphs and nits. Similarly, Buddhist monks shave to promote humility (and cleanliness).

However, hair length is not necessarily a factor in infestation itself. It is, in fact, social behaviour that explains why louse rates in boys were lower in the 1940s, when hair was worn short and shaking hands was the customary way of greeting. In the 1970s, when the fashion was for longer styles, a more casual physical approach was culturally more acceptable.

The 'Mohican' (or Mohawk) cut popularly adopted by punks is thought to have originated in Africa and the Americas as a way of managing head lice. The hair behind the ears and at the nape of the neck, where nits are mostly laid, are the areas subject to rigorous shaving while the 'comb' on top is kept long in order to aid the combing out of live insects who gravitate towards the centre parting.

WHY DO WE SCRATCH?

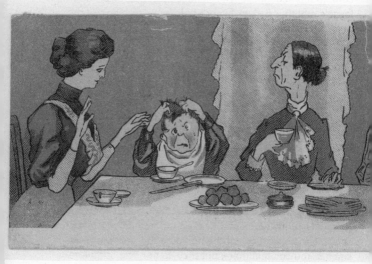

"You rude boy, how dare you scratch your head at the table."

"Well, they started at me first."

It's not the pain of the bite that makes us scratch. Everyone from Aristotle onwards knew that louse bites were nothing (mind you, he also thought that people with head lice were less prone to headaches).

Researchers feeding laboratory lice on the backs of their hands also feel no pain. You can undertake this same experiment in the comfort of your own home next time you comb out a head louse. The slender sucking tube of the louse's mouth is a sleek hypodermic fang, nothing like the mosquito's dagger.

Over time, louse saliva can cause irritation in the skin and this rash can sometimes itch. But the real shivering sensation that gets the finger nails rasping across the head is just the head lice moseying about in the hair.

Here's another experiment to try. Touch just a single hair on your own head and you can feel it immediately. It tickles. But run your fingers through your hair and even though thousands of strands are being stimulated in the same way, you do not feel tickled a thousandfold. If anything, the greater the stimulus, the less the sensation.

There's a good biological reason for this. You do not want to be constantly distracted by the wind tickling your head, so large-scale rustlings of the hair do not fire off warning signals. You can feel them, but they do not itch. Stimulate just one or two hairs — as a louse does tiptoeing across the scalp – and the tingling is suddenly intense.

And why do we scratch the tingle? Because scratching is one of the best ways to damage, or kill, a head louse. Second only to combing, really.

Is Scratching Catching?

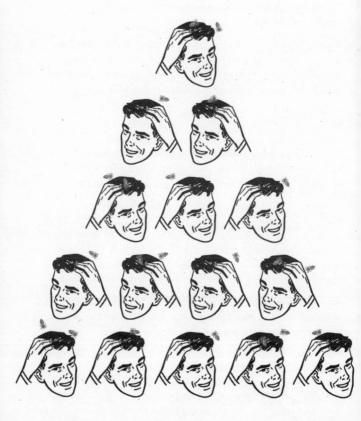

According to one louse writer in the 1950s, we do not scratch enough. He reasoned that if we scratched more, we'd kill more head lice. He blamed the 'social taboo that exists in many circles against scratching'. Part of this he put down to elaborate hair styles which may prevent 'savage man and civilised woman' from scratching their heads.

Scratching, like blushing and yawning, is catching. There is another good biological reason for this. Blushing is the silent human way of communicating agreement: 'yes, I agree, this is embarrassing, isn't it?' or 'yes, I sympathise with your situation' or even, if romantic novels are to be believed, 'yes, I love you too'. Likewise, yawning shows a general group agreement that everyone is tired, so there's no danger from squabbling, fighting or killing tonight.

Copying someone else's scratching is a good defence tactic. The reasoning goes something like this:

1 that person is scratching so they are likely to have lice;

2 they are near me so I am likely to have caught lice even if I don't know it yet;

3 I'll get scratching now and squash the vermin before they have a chance to breed;

4 ooh, that feels good.

'Break their legs, they can't lay eggs'.

Head lice cannot heal themselves, so having a leg pulled off by being scratched is fatal for a louse.

CHEMICAL WARFARE

The head louse was heard to complain
That a chemist had poisoned his brain.
The cause of his sorrow
Was *para-dichloro-
Diphenyltrichloroethane*

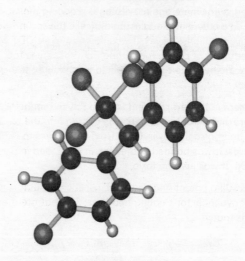

With apologies to Dr D.D. Perrin, professor in the Department
of Medical Chemistry of the Australian National University,
whose original version mentioned a mosquito.

Combing, grooming and nit-picking are so old-fashioned – all very eighteenth century. The nineteenth wasn't much better, ridding yourself and your children of head lice meant smearing heads with paraffin, naphthalene (moth balls), turpentine (paint thinners), carbolic acid and all manner of corrosive and poisonous gloop.

This is the modern world and what we need is a modern solution. That modern solution arrived in 1939, when Swiss chemist Paul Müller was tinkering with a colourless and almost odourless white crystalline substance called dichlorodiphenyltrichloroethane. He discovered it was quite the most poisonous thing for insects. Almost overnight it became the biggest and best insecticide on the planet: DDT.

DDT revolutionised delousing. And although it was also sprayed everywhere against disease-spreading mosquitoes and crop pests, its use against body lice in the second world war saved millions of lives. It wasn't long before DDT was the treatment of choice for getting rid of head lice too. And it worked very well ⚊ for a bit. Then something got in the way.

Elsewhere in the environment, sprayed by the tonne from tractors and aeroplanes, DDT was getting into the food chain and poisoning everything from honeybees to Honey Buzzards. It was banned in the USA in 1972 and in Britain in 1984. It was just too toxic.

DDT is still a potent and powerful insecticide, but it is no longer available for treating head lice. So what are the options today?

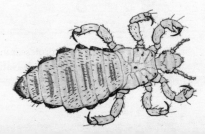

POTIONS
AND
POISONS

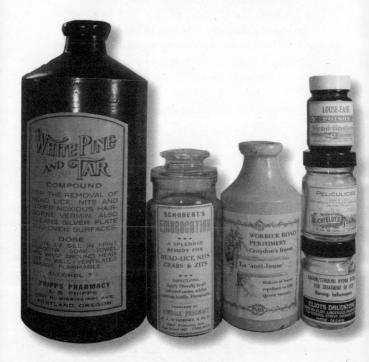

If you take your head lice to the doctor, he or she is likely to offer you chemical treatment. After all, prescribing drugs is what doctors do. What you are given depends on where you live. In the UK, at the time of writing, the 'official' National Health Service treatments were a variety of branded liquids to apply to the head. These will contain either:

- dimeticone
- isopropyl myristate and cyclomethicone
- coconut, anise and ylang ylang
- malathion

Don't be confused by the synthetic chemical-sounding names of three of them and the plant-named one in the middle: this is just down to the branding preferences of the pharmaceutical companies, who have plumped either for a high-tech scientific route or a friendly back-to-nature version.

Everything named above is an insecticide and they will kill lice. Or they will kill some of them. And there's the rub. No chemical can claim to be 100% effective. Not killing all of the lice just makes for a bigger headache.

We all lead busy lives and head louse treatments are often rushed. Anti-louse shampoos are smeared on but washed off too soon, or not repeated often enough. A few lice aren't killed. They are the tougher ones, the ones who are slightly resistant to the insecticidal poisoning action. They survive and they have louselings which are tough too. Just like a breeding programme to give bigger, better and tougher farm animals, insecticide treatments are creating tougher insecticide-resistant head lice▾

New chemicals come along, but each time the lice outwit us. Some always survive. Better get out that old-fashioned comb. Oh look. The final option for the UK doctor is to prescribe a 'Bug Buster®' comb.

Lotions and *Shampoos*

Hedrin ~ **Full Marks** ~ Vosene Kids ~ Escenti Children's Tea Tree ~ *Dr Johnsons Repellent Head Lice Shampoo* ~ **Lyclear** ~ Ginesis Lice Trap Shampoo ~ Lanes Tea Tree Shampoo ~ Lice Blaster ~ RID Lice Killing Shampoo ~ *Tisserand Tea Lemon & Rosemary Shampoo* ~ B3 Blitz Headlice Shampoo ~ Boots Pharmaceutical Head Lice Remover Mousse ~ **Liceadex Lice & Nit Removal Gel** ~ Nitty Gritty Headlice Solution ~ *Head-On Aromatherapy Lice Targeting Shampoo* ~ Healthaid Tea Tree Shampoo ~ NitWits All-in-One ~ A-Lices Scalp & Body Hygiene Shampoo ~ **What Nits!** ~ *Picksan Lice Stop Anti Lice Shampoo* ~ Pyrifoam Shampoo ~ Lice Shield 2-in-1 Shampoo & Conditioner ~ Lice Out Lice Immobilizing Gel ~ *Circle of Friends Lice Defense Shampoo* ~ **Derbac** ~ Lyderm Cream ~ Lincin ~ Zippity-Doo's Shampoo Lice Prevention ~ *Lice and Nit Eliminating Natural Mousse with Foam* ~ Eco Kid Prevent Kit ~ Parasidose Extra Strength Lice Shampoo ~ Mediker Anti Lice Treatment ~ *Naturado Organic Anti Lice Solution* ~ **Nix Cream Rinse** ~ Vogel Riddance ~ Electric Blue Head Lice Cream ~ Naturally Does It ~ Nelson's Nice 'N Clear ~ **Cetaphil** ~ Ovide Solution ~ Lice Attack … *ad infinitum*

'I was amazed by the choice of products in our local independent pharmacy … even the pharmacist seemed a bit bewildered and kept saying that it all depended on how much I wanted to spend.'

Jonathan, Maidstone

Getting rid of head lice is big business: the shampoos and lotions (not to mention repellent sprays, gels and mousses, and kits, combs and gadgets) on the shelves at the chemist and in your supermarket are not cheap. Apparently, the 'head lice industry' is worth £33.5 million in the UK alone. The cynic may argue that if these products worked, ultimately there wouldn't be an industry. Others suggest that head lice will always find ways to adapt and as their host is replenished, a fresh set of heads to infest appears with every generation. Basically, so long as the human race exists, head lice will continue to drive us crazy as we try to eradicate them. And they'll make us poorer too.

In the chemist you will find:

- **topical insecticides,** which usually include permethrin. Head lice are increasingly resistant to these drugs as a result of genetic mutation;
- **cleansers,** these skin-care products claim to suffocate head lice;
- **over-the-counter non-pesticide preparations,** these usually contain the essential oils (such as rosemary, tea tree and citronella) that have natural antiseptic properties;
- **egg removal shampoos,** this kind of product claims to 'help loosen lice';
- **sprays,** these coat the hair, therefore acting as a repellent;
- **mousses and gels,** these are like lotions, but thicker.

But which to choose?

Oils: Essential, Aromatherapy and Cooking

Oils for your shopping list that some claim to be useful in pursuit of the itch.

tea tree oil – perennial favourite and answer to all the world's ills;

peppermint oil – apparently contains a high concentration of natural pesticides;

lavender oil – thought to disinfect the scalp and skin;

catnip oil – also used as a mosquito repellent;

erigeron oil – known as fleabane in the USA;

neem oil – an apparently natural pesticide;

rosemary oil – used to obtain softer, smoother hair;

karanja oil – often used in pet care for the treatment of fleas, mange and scabies;

citronella oil – a common insect repellent;

cedar oil – extracted from the bark of the tree, this oil has been used as an insect repellent for hundreds of years

'I went on holiday with some dear friends, good company in every way except for two things. Firstly, they insisted on reading aloud the Harry Potter novels to their children on the beach; secondly, they also nit-combed them on the beach – with olive oil. I was dubious but seeing as I had to comb my children if theirs were in the thrall of infestation, it seemed rude – if not disparaging – not to use the oil too. So there we sat, tugging combs through hair knotted with sea salt, with a persistent marine breeze playing havoc with the tissues, unable to tell what was nit, what was louse and what was sand. I don't know who was having the hardest time of it – Harry as he battled Voldemort or us as we attempted to keep grip on combs greasy with extra virgin while encrusted with most of the Normandy coastline.'

Andrea, Anerley

Plain old combing with some kind of slippery base is still the most efficient treatment for removing lice and nits. It is a method that has been used for millennia. However, alternative therapies, folklore and some scientists maintain that certain oils also have properties useful in the eradication of head lice▾

The problem with using oil, of course, is that it is difficult to remove once you have finished with it. Various Internet sites recommend coating the hair with baking powder after treatment and then rinsing off. Make sure you set aside plenty of time, not to mention ingredients!

With its delicious camphorous scent, tea tree oil from Australia was used by indigenous aborigines to treat skin maladies and colds and certainly the limited modern research conducted has revealed antibacterial, antifungal and antiseptic qualities in this wonder juice. Bought by the gallon by those looking for a natural product, one that's organic (therefore, safe?), cheap and most importantly, one that does all the hard work effortlessly, it is the favourite of yummy mummies everywhere. You can smell them coming a mile off.

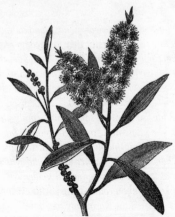

Historical Treatments

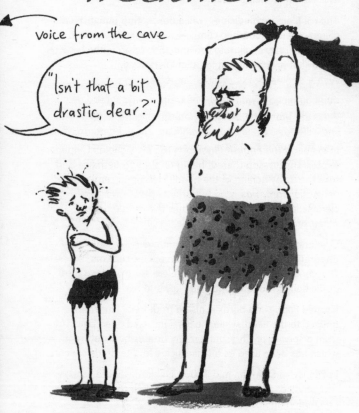

Head lice have been a problem
for thousands of years.

S tavesacre, sometimes known as a lousewort, is a species of larkspur cultivated in Southern Europe. It was known to both the Greeks and the Romans, prized during medieval times as a herb and, according to *The Modern Herbal*, as a parasiticide. Poisonous, it features in many ancient recipes and recommendations.

Ancient Chinese medicine – while advocating patience and diligence with a bamboo comb ➝ recommends stemona root. Boil it, strain, allow to cool and then apply to the head, which should be wrapped overnight in a towel.

During the 1600s, Native Americans boiled down mesquite and combined it with mud. The mixture was spread on the scalp and left in place for two days in order to destroy head lice▾

In his book *The English Physitian* (1652), Nicholas Culpeper wrote, 'The Hyssop thereof being anointed killeth lice and take the away itching of the head'. Hyssop, a semi-woody aromatic plant, was used to purify temples and cleanse lepers. Hyssop oil contains the ketone thujone, a neurotoxin, and pinocamphone.

Oregano also has antiseptic and antiparasitic qualities apparently useful in the eradication of head lice and scabies. Dioscorides, a Greek physician in Nero's army, noted that garlic boiled with oregano killed lice and bed bugs.

Horned Poppy and borax is also a traditional 'cure' when applied to the head, while the Persians used dried petals from a species of Chrysanthemum, producing Pyrethrum, which has been used as an insecticide for hundreds of years.

In Pennsylvania in the mid 1800s, children went to school with small caches of brimstone tied at their throats as a precaution against lice.

A mixture of mercury, hog fat and mutton suet rubbed on the head is cited as a suggestion to destroy body lice in the 1881 *Household Cyclopedia*.

Alternative Remedies *and* Home Brews

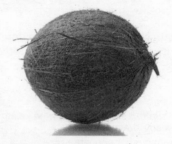

From an Internet Chatroom

'When I was young, I had lice in my hair. My mom put virgin coconut oil in my hair. This hardens below 24°C. The oil hardened in my hair and the lice died.'

The same forum officially pronounces that 'living lice eggs tend to be pale white' and 'dead lice eggs are orangeish'. If this is what you believe, go back to the very beginning of this book and start reading it all over again▾

For instance, certain Internet sites claim that coconut oil is not only the ideal slippery base for removing nits, but that it has properties that help penetrate the exoskeletons of the lice. One in particular insists that use of coconut oil in conjunction with another, such as peppermint oil or eucalyptus oil, will stun the lice. Use of a shower cap once the scalp is coated, they say, will then prevent the lice trying to escape by 'jumping off'.

From our blog

Lily Says…

Today, three beautiful teenage girls are lounging around talking about getting nits. Lily says, 'My mum once counted a hundred head lice off my head in just 15 minutes!' The other two find this outrageous and gasp, hands clapped to their lipsticked mouths in disgust. 'And then,' Lily continues, 'she made me bend down and sit for an hour with my head in a bucket of vinegar!' And the three of them absolutely explode with laughter at the ridiculous image this conjures. They are still shedding tears 10 minutes later. I am still giggling too, but more out of disbelief. That someone so lovely and intelligent could have a parent so very ill-informed.

While vinegar is a fairly common 'alternative' remedy, there are plenty of other recipes and other home-brewed solutions out there that many sufferers are still convinced really work.

'Acetic acid or vinegar is still popular owing to the belief that it loosens the cement attaching the egg to the hair. It has been known for years that this is not so, and that even after several days exposure, the cement is not dissolved.' P. A. Buxton, 1939.

More Alternatives

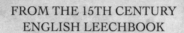

FROM THE 15TH CENTURY
ENGLISH LEECHBOOK

FOR NITS IN THE HEAD,

~ make lye of wild nept (bryony) and
therewith wash your head

~ take quicklime or piment and make powder
of them and mix with vinegar and
anoint the head with it

~ take seawater or else also brine and wash
your head and it shall destroy them

~ take juice of a herb that is called blight
and anoint your head with it, both lice
and nits shall fall away

~ take a broad list (a ribbon of fabric)
and anoint one side with fresh grease
mingled with quicksilver (mercury) and
spread on it a powder of lichen, and
wear it henceforth

Marmalade. Mr Jones tells me a remedy using this exists. I think he may have dreamed it. We have nits on the brain.

Vaseline. Apply to the head for eight hours overnight under a shower cap and bingo, the next day it promises to provide you with a hat full of dead lice.

Kerosene. *Don't try this at home, folks!* However, once upon a time ➤ and until quite recently ➤ this was a recommended solution to lice infestation, especially in the Antipodes.

Hair dye. A fairly drastic solution to an infestation is dying the hair. It is said that the strong chemicals used by professional stylists are potent enough to kill live lice. The dry heat from a hairdryer hood may also be effective. Prepare for a long afternoon and an eye-watering bill. But you will look beautiful.

Vinegar. This recipe comes from an Internet site. Add 30 drops of lavender oil to 25cl good (!) wine vinegar, macerate for seven days, shake vigorously and rub on to the head. Use regularly as (apparently) 'lice hate the smell'.

Mayonnaise. Use a full-fat variety as apparently this is more effective. I am also informed that you need to keep it on your head for eight hours, although 'not overnight' as mayonnaise 'turns rancid after a few hours out of the fridge'. The combined properties of the dressing are supposed to suffocate the live lice.

Wood chips (yes...). Boil 'em in water for 20 minutes and pour the water on your head – when it has cooled, silly...

Apply and wait for the old wives to be proved correct.

THE NIT NURSE

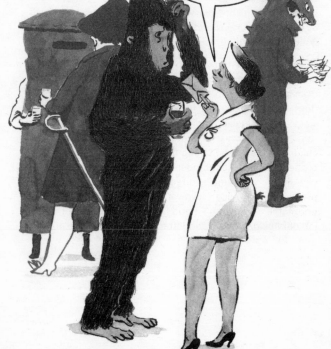

Until the late 1980s, the 'nit nurse' ➤ a term first coined in the 1940s – was a common presence in primary schools. In fact, these were designated school nurses given the job of lining up the children to check heads once or twice a year in the hope of detecting infestation. If a case was confirmed, the pupil in question would often be sent home with the dreaded brown envelope.

The demise of the nit nurse came when the NHS was reorganised in 1974. The policy of having a specific nurse attached to a school changed to a more general community role. A qualified nurse would be based at a GP's practice or health centre and would visit a number of schools in the area to advise on all sorts of matters, oversee vaccinations and to raise awareness of health issues in general.

There have been many campaigns in recent years to 'bring back the nit nurse'. Those against argue that there is no evidence that nits and lice were any less prevalent in the days of the sick bay and brown envelope. As they see it, a single quick glance at one head in a thousand is unlikely to result in a successful find, but it does ensure that some children are exposed to stigmatisation. Those in favour of the revival argue that identifying repeat offenders will 'shame' the families affected into dealing with the problem of head lice. However, as far as we know – and as adaptable as they are – head lice are still not put off the job of infestation by a stiff letter from the nit nurse.

Gadgets, *Zappers* and *Other* Methods

'I bought one of those electrical louse buster gadgets online. A small charge kills the lice when it is trapped between alternating negative and positive tines. Armed with my prod, heeding all warnings to use the thing on dry hair only and convinced that they weren't sufferers of epilepsy or fitted with cardiac pacemakers, I lined up my children and began the process of electrical annihilation. The first candidate, my short-haired five-year-old found it tickly – fascinating, even – but we didn't catch anything

The second, my middle daughter, fidgeted terribly so I wasn't sure how well I had swept her head. With wet combing you can at least see where you've been, but we saw nothing. Finally, my nearly teenage son capitulated. Just when I thought we were making progress – I'm pretty certain I fried at least two live insects as the gadget stopped buzzing both times – he too began to wriggle whenever I pressed the button. After the third attempt to get him to keep still, I realised the problem: the rubber coating had already worn off a couple of the tines and I was delivering neat wee electric shocks to his scalp! I chucked it away immediately and we have stuck with a plain old metal comb ever since. But we still have a laugh about the day Mummy zapped Harry!'

Caroline, West Sussex

ROLL UP, ROLL UP

... witness all **VARIETY** of **INNOVATION** and **MEDICATION**
dedicated to the cause of head louse **ERADICATION**
(and often, the making of **MONEY**, thereof ...)

ELECTRONIC LICE COMBS

Usually battery powered, these work by administering an
electrical **CHARGE** to the trapped **LOUSE**.

ELECTRONIC LICE DETECTORS AND REMOVERS

As above lice combs, for your **DELECTATION** and for the
ILLUSION of choice, but with different product name.

HEATED-AIR LOUSE BLOWERS

These work on the **PRINCIPLE** of heat and wind
VELOCITY drying out the adult insect, as it requires
a moist environment to **SURVIVE**.

ONLINE LICE COMBING SERVICES

Pick up the **PHONE** or send an **EMAIL** and they come round
and do the hard work for you – **FOR A FEE**.

YOUTUBE

There are **VIDEOS** online should you need to
watch **ERADICATION** in **ACTION**.

Nit-B-Gone,
Nits Away,
I Can't Believe
it's Not Nits!

Removing head lice is one thing. At least they can be combed away. But removing nits is another ⚫ remember that excellent nit glue pages 20–1? Not that there is any real need to remove nits. They are already empty, they cannot hatch and they do no harm.

They might look a bit unsightly, however, and the ill-informed no-nit policies of some schools have created a 'need' to remove them. So all manner of nit-removing chemicals have been developed.

But do they work? Until now, all we had to go on was personal testimony and vague anecdote. Vinegar has been paraded about for its supposed nit-loosening ability for years. But what strength should be used? How long should you leave it on? And what type should you use? White wine, cider, malt or balsamic? There is now a way to tell.

Cambridge phthirapterist Ian Burgess has developed a nit 'slideability' testing machine. It's an ingenious device. A single hair, with nit attached, is threaded into a tiny tube only just wide enough to take it, until the nit becomes lodged in the narrow opening at one end. At the other end, the hair is attached to a small turning drum, which gradually applies increasing pulling power until the nit starts to slip along the hair shaft. The exact amount of pull needed to rip off the nit can now be measured with precise accuracy.

So how did vinegar do? Indeed, how did the specialist nit-loosening preparations do? Did they make it easier to pull the nits off the hair strands? No, they didn't. They had no effect whatsoever other than to lubricate the hair shaft just like water or over-the-counter hair conditioner. Burgess's conclusion? That 'so-called "nit-removing" products have no effect'. There you have it ⚫ from the phthirapterist's mouth.

How Do Animals Cope with Lice?

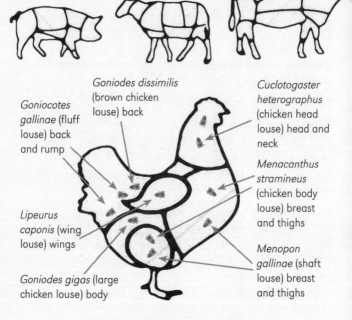

Goniocotes gallinae (fluff louse) back and rump

Goniodes dissimilis (brown chicken louse) back

Cuclotogaster heterographus (chicken head louse) head and neck

Lipeurus caponis (wing louse) wings

Menacanthus stramineus (chicken body louse) breast and thighs

Goniodes gigas (large chicken louse) body

Menopon gallinae (shaft louse) breast and thighs

Chickens, it seems, have more than their fair share of lice.

With only three louse species to contend with (see pages 102–3), we are at the easy end of the infestation spectrum. Since they are at the centre of a multi-billion dollar industry throughout the world, we know lots about poultry lice. Poor old Mrs Chicken has to cope with seven species of louse. Battery chickens are not very good at ridding themselves of lice, but that may be something to do with the fact they are inbred, crowded, cramped, in unnatural conditions and fed too much.

Grooming is a natural behaviour displayed by most birds and mammals, and it works. We know this from observations of animals unable to groom. Sick or senile cats and dogs have much higher louse infestations. Birds with damaged beaks always have more lice than healthy nestmates. Laboratory mice keep their lice at least contained to the neck region, unless prevented from grooming using their legs; in which case the lice spread all over the body.

Birds go to great lengths to keep their feathers free of vermin, including rolling in dust, bathing in puddles and anointing themselves with ants. The ants they choose are not stinging varieties, but those that spray formic acid out of their back ends. Experiments have shown that the acid can play a role in killing lice, but the main benefit seems to be keeping the birds' feathers in good condition.

Higher primates groom each other and the image of a mother ape nit-picking parasites from the fluffy nape of her young is a familiar heart-warming reminder of just how intelligent and caring our primate relatives are.

'It's lice, Jim, but not as we know it.'

Combs – Up There with the Wheel and the Mobile Phone?

As a piece of design, the humble comb has withstood the test of time, and continues to withstand the test of lice.

Remember, you are not combing lice out of the luxuriant hair: they are not like monkeys swinging through the trees. You are scraping them *off the scalp*. Dig deep and pretend you are hunting for wild boar running among the tree trunks.

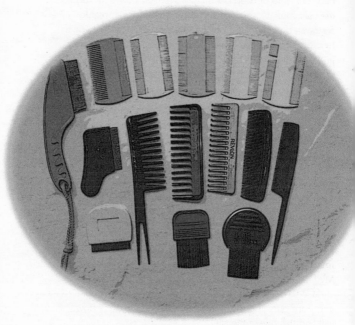

You have to be a dedicated nit-picker to build up a collection as useful as mine.

From our blog

The Louse Hunter

The basic design of a nit comb is near perfection – tight tines and something to hold. They have been found among Egyptian tomb goods destined for the afterlife (it wouldn't do to be itchy for eternity, eh?) and in caves excavated in Israel dating to the first century BC. Fashioned from various types of ivory and wood, they have also been recovered from shipwrecks like that of the *Mary Rose*, Henry VIII's beloved yet ill-fated warship. Rats, scurvy, Spaniards and head lice ➤ those were the days!

First, the wide-toothed is arguably the most important comb in the collection. No, it doesn't capture any beasts – not intentionally, anyway – but combined with conditioner, it conquers the initial tangles that make the job of the louse hunter so tough.

Next is the double-sided plastic job. Ordinarily, it's not very useful at all – it has no grip and the tines aren't close enough – but if you have a small child, this is *their* comb. I find that Barbies, contrary to my usual opinion of the miniature dolly birds, come into their own here: they can be combed too (doesn't work on Transformers, however).

Also available is a long-toothed branded steel comb which promises to rid the entire universe of head lice for a mere ten quid. My friend Sally swears by hers although I am yet to catch a live louse in its kinks. I have also found the grip awkward. But I do find this comb can hoik out a nit or two when all other combs have failed.

If I ever see a nit comb that purports to be better than all the rest, I am cautious. After all, if the design ain't broke, why fix it? My favourite is a small white one with metal teeth and a rough surface to hold on to. This is the most vital piece of equipment in my armoury. It grips, it traps. When my ship goes down, they will find this one in the silt.

Louse (and Comb) Timeline

8000 BC   Nit identified on a human hair in Brazil.

3000 BC   Nits on an Egyptian mummy.

430 AD   Herodotus describes how priests took precautions against lice infestation.

350 BC   Aristotle writes theory of how lice occur.

72 AD   A comb with a louse attached at Hadrian's Wall, Cumbria.

79 AD   A louse egg on the head of a female who perished when Mount Vesuvius erupted.

4th, 5th and 6th century   Combs with lice in tombs in Egypt.

16th century   The Mary Rose sinks in the Solent with nit combs among the salvage.

17th century   Bevelled combs from the Navajo people, SW USA.

Hurrah for the humble comb!

17th century	New England Puritans use wooden nit combs in Massachusetts, USA.
1758	Start of modern scientific name for human louse, *Pediculus humanus*, coined by Swedish naturalist Carl Linnaeus.
1767	Linnaeus's compatriot Charles De Geer, distinguishes head louse as a different species, naming it *Pediculus capitis*.
1842	Henry Denny writes *Monographia Anoplurum Britanniae*, first major monograph on lice in English.
1939	Insecticidal properties of DDT discovered.
1977	Permethrin manufactured as head louse treatment.
1995	Evidence of pyrethroid resistance grows∗
2005	Comb and conditioner elimination method found to be 57% successful, compared to 13% using synthetic chemical based insecticide preparations.
2007	Metal-tined brand-name comb tested against a normal plastic comb shows a greater efficacy in removing nits.

RACIST BUGS?

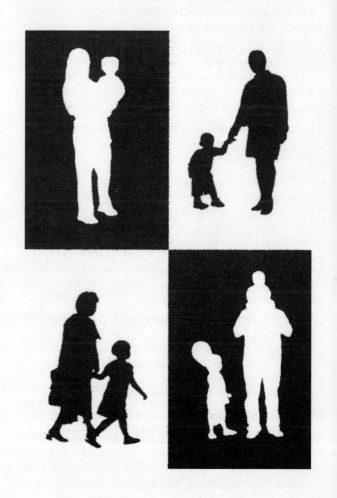

Y ou will often hear tales that Afro-Caribbean kids don't get nits. Nonsense, of course. But how about the claim that they are *less prone* to head lice than their white-skinned classmates? There may be some truth in this. Not much truth, just *some* truth.

Even the oldest textbooks state: 'no human race is without lice, or immune to them'. Lice have tormented humans throughout their history, on every continent, in every era. But it is true that in Europe and North America, head lice are *sometimes* less common on Afro-Caribbean heads.

It has nothing to do with skin colour, diet, clothes, religious belief, family background or distant racial homeland. It has everything to do with hair type.

Tiny head lice are supremely adapted to live in hair ... *of a particular size*. It's all to do with the size of those powerful hair-gripping claws (see pages 28–9). Soft, wavy blonde hair is very thin, about 17–50µm (thousandths of a millimetre) in diameter. Afro-Caribbean hair is much thicker, 60–180µm. Of course there is a complete range of hair sizes, from one extreme to the other, but in a predominantly white population, most lice will be adapted to live amongst the smaller diameter hairs of the majority.

This will not stop lice moving from blonde head to black (or brunette, redhead, grey or blue-rinse), but it may mean that once arrived, they will not move around quite so easily on the scalp. The lice may not be able to attach their eggs so carefully to the thicker hairs. They may get dislodged, or damaged, more easily. They may not do so well.

It's no use being complacent, though. Everyone can get head lice ◄ whatever their skin colour, whatever their hair type.

MASS NIT-BUSTING

There are companies and charities → often approved by the NHS → that advocate so-called 'bug-busting days'. Trademarked combs are supplied to schools along with literature explaining why the entire school roll should use the combs on a particular day.

The laudable argument is that if schools synchronise their mass combing, infestation levels will be reduced along with healthcare costs. Health inequalities will also be addressed and by using the 'whole school' method, the social stigma attached to the issue is also minimised.

In Denmark, they have had a Great Louse Day since 2002. Elsewhere, there have been calls for a national nit day where everybody with hair gets the detection comb out and goes hunting. Ultimately, though, hard work followed up by routine is the key to eradication within the community.

'We haven't had many problems for a few years, although I shouldn't speak too soon. But at my son's previous school there were such problems with head lice that the PTA paid for head louse combs to be given to every child in the school – a brilliant idea! I still have the same comb and at the first whisper of head lice it comes out and is used for a week or so, whether we find any or not. I have to admit I'm not sure I would have bothered to get one if I hadn't been given one. My son hates it, obviously, but I'm sure everyone knows that it's easier if you use it along with conditioner.'

Gill, Nunhead

'Our school sent each pupil home with a fluorescent plastic comb and strict instructions to comb our child's head on the 31st of the coming month. I didn't mind doing this as the problem has been so bad that I felt that any action was better than doing nothing. The trouble is some parents thought it was a bit of a joke, others questioned whether the school should be spending money on things like this when it had a shortage of PE equipment and books, and I saw one woman just drop the pack in the bin. I felt that I had done my bit by sticking to the date and that nobody could accuse my family of complacency.'

Lois, Southwark

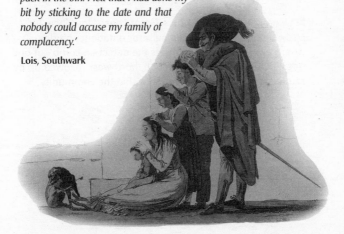

The Little Nit *Timeline*

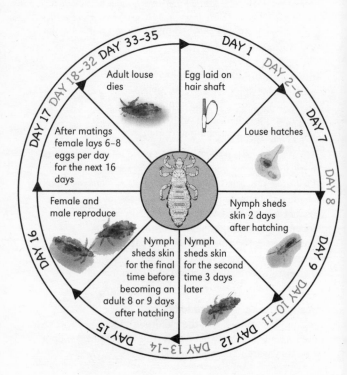

DAY 33–35 — Adult louse dies

DAY 1 — Egg laid on hair shaft

DAY 2–6 / DAY 7 — Louse hatches

DAY 18–32 — After matings female lays 6–8 eggs per day for the next 16 days

DAY 8 — Nymph sheds skin 2 days after hatching

DAY 17 / DAY 16 — Female and male reproduce

DAY 9 / DAY 10–11 / DAY 12 — Nymph sheds skin for the second time 3 days later

DAY 15 — Nymph sheds skin for the final time before becoming an adult 8 or 9 days after hatching

DAY 13–14

Elbow Grease and Routine

The Justine Crow Method

Every Tuesday, I combed my children's heads in the bath. Head lice aren't particularly averse to Tuesdays but it was hair-washing night, simple as that. I always had bottles and cups for them to play with as well as a plentiful supply of cheap conditioner, inexpensive tissues and a cup full of combs. The bath was important because it meant the kids couldn't escape. I combed as close to the scalp as possible without scratching it, and inspected and wiped the comb every single swipe.

On a good Tuesday, I found nothing. Sometimes, however, I'd fish out a couple. This meant I'd comb again on Thursday or Friday and always on the following Tuesday. My rationale was that if I combed every week without fail, regardless of detection, I would keep the problem to a minimum. We had a 'count to twenty' rule — after 10 or 15 minutes combing, we would count every stroke. If we found nothing after 20 strokes, we would stop. If we found a nit or a louse, the count went back to zero.

Infestation always seemed to occur when there was a break in this routine. Yes, the children yelled and yes, they hated it, but they grew used to it. They never knew a time when they weren't combed weekly.

SHIPBUILDING

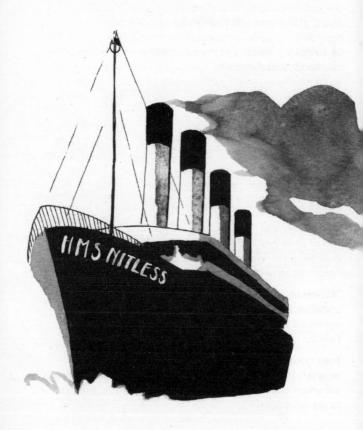

At the beginning of the 20th century, head lice were seen as the scourge of working class children, and 'correction' ✶ applied almost like a punishment ✶ was one of the ambitions of the education system. This marked the beginning of the 'nit letter', sent home with the embarrassed child to the upset parents. The School Board of Glasgow was just as rigorous as any other in recording its pupils' lousiness. Their statistics now give us an intriguing insight into the relationship between poverty and head louse numbers.

The principal industry of Glasgow at the time was shipbuilding, and there were lean times as well as productive ones. Although unemployment figures were not officially recorded then, there is a good relationship between head lice and ship production (which was well recorded).

Between 1910 and 1930, whenever there was a drop in shipbuilding, with the attendant loss of employment to its workers and hardship for their families, there was an increase in head lice. The peak of louse infestation came two or three years into the recession, when times were at their toughest. When ship construction resumed and the hardships were lifted, the lice declined.

This association of head lice with working class deprivation ended in the late 1940s, as chemical control methods appeared and the National Health Service at last offered help for free.

Even more striking, since 1976, head louse infestations have left the urban poor and become the affliction of rural, suburban and middle-class children. You're never too posh to get head lice✶

POPULATION DYNAMICS

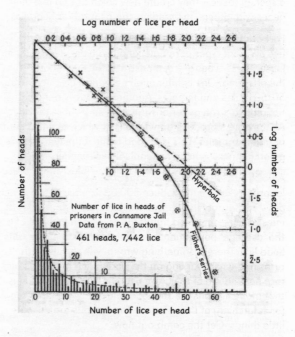

Log number of lice per head

Number of heads

Log number of heads

Number of lice in heads of prisoners in Cannamore Jail
Data from P. A. Buxton
461 heads, 7,442 lice

Hyperbola

Fisher's series

Number of lice per head

Understanding louse population dynamics requires a fair amount of maths. The lice don't bother with calculations though, they just get on with it.

Head lice are niftily active and it is easily possible for a single louse to spend the day visiting several different heads. As phthirapterist John Maunder puts it brilliantly, head lice are not castaways marooned on separate islands, but an actively intermingling community living on an archipelago.

The most adventurous lice are newly mated females, who will swap heads at a moment's notice. This is the perfect dispersal tactic – they create new colonies and mix their genes with others. In-breeding can be fatal for head lice.

Part of this is down to the fact that there are (at least) five different types of female, and two types of male head louse. These types are demonstrated by the sex ratios of the offspring. One combination of mating produces around 50/50 males and females. Another produces only males: not a good strategy for ensuring the survival of the species. All the others produce populations in which females greatly outnumber males. This is a good tactic if the females are to go on dangerous head-to-head colonisation journeys*

An average louse lives for about 30 days (60 in the laboratory) and can produce 300 eggs, each of which can grow to maturity in 20 days. Despite horrendous tales of infestations containing hundreds or even thousands of lice, the 'average' population on an infested head is 10–20 head lice. There is something wrong with this, though. It turns out, when working on the population mathematics, that not enough of them are nymphs. The explanation is that many nymphs die young, damaged by the grooming (or scratching) of their victims. The nymphs are delicate little things. Get the comb out now.

What Would Happen If We Did Nothing?

Apparently in the 'Middle Ages', the election of the local burgomaster in Hurdenburg, Sweden, was governed by the wanderings of a louse. Candidates for this mayor-type position sat down and rested their beards on a table. A louse was released into the centre of the table and the owner of the beard first honoured by the louse's occupancy was elected.

It all seems just a little odd, though. In fact, this 'fact' arose from a second-hand report in a book published in 1865. It has been repeated almost word for word ever since, however, and has spread to such an extent that this is now the only 'fact' known about the town or city of Hurdenburg.

No one knows where is Hurdenburg is. It does not exist on modern maps. It may be Hedberg, in the Arvidsjaur Kommun, near Norrbottens. Wherever, it's too similar-sounding to 'headbug', surely. Or maybe that's how the place got its name?

And what could be the rationale behind such a bizarre protocol? Was the elder with the longest beard (probably the oldest person there) reasoned to have the greatest experience and lore? There is still a lot more research to do before we can accept this ridiculous piece of historical hearsay.

From our blog

My chum Kaye has a Facebook friend who put out the question: 'My child has come home with nits, any suggestions?' 'She's a natural Mother Earth type,' Kaye reported and my heart sank.

There were many, many Mother Earth types at the excellent festival I went to with my offspring a couple of Julys ago. It seems the English summer, though cruel to everyone else, was kind to us and we had three days of sunshine and grubby pleasure sitting in the grass, drinking beer in the afternoon ⟵ me that is, not my children. We wandered around the entertainment stalls, therapy tents and daft workshops and listened to a lot of live music. One afternoon, the main field was full of dancing adults and sheepish children embarrassed by their parents and a friend introduced me to an arty sort she thought I might get along with.

She was indeed interesting so we chatted and watched and supped from cans. Eventually I couldn't help but giggle and point out several children who were mucking around among the revellers dressed in oversized T-shirts, sporting long matted plaits and bare feet. I was amused because every so often, they stopped and gave their heads a good scratch.

'Hah! Just look at those kids going behind their ears like hound dogs! They are absolutely riddled!', I chortled.

And my new acquaintance laughed and agreed with me and we carried on. It was only later that I saw her giving them some money to go and get themselves something to eat.

So, I asked Kaye, what was the advice that came back on Facebook? 'All kinds,' Kaye replied but ultimately the Mother Earth type had decided to 'let nature take its course'.

'When it comes to nits, you cannot make like an ostrich and bury your head in the sand.'

HOLIDAYS

That holiday packing list in full

- Nit comb
- Conditioner
- Tissues
- Er, that's it ...

'We had a holiday when the whole family was full of nits and ended up passing them on to the other two families staying with us. In the end, we had a mass de-nitting event in the courtyard beside the old French farmhouse we'd rented, with all chairs outside and 11 kids and six adults all being combed. Very picturesque it was. Mind you, the French conditioner was rubbish: too posh and not slippery enough.'

Becky, Greenwich

From our blog

Can the Fleas Come Too?

Why not take the whole family on holiday, insects and all? C'mon, you haven't lived until you've shuffled around Super U in Northern France wondering what the difference is between *shampooing* and *après shampooing*, apart from the *après*. Given that the price of the latter is often double the former, you'd safely assume that the 'after' gunk is conditioner. It is, but not as we know it.

I never thought I'd hear myself say how lucky we are to have supermarkets as we do in the UK, although you'll be pleased to know I've made it a rule of life never to cross the threshold of a certain chain, even during a nit emergency (and that includes the French equivalent with a remarkably similar *trois pour deux* philosophy). But we *are* lucky because we get a whole aisle of conditioners to choose from, whereas the French get precisely two bottles of *après shampooing*. And the one you put in your *chariot* (I love that: 'bring me my chariot!'; 'Crikey, she's off her chariot...') is mysteriously inept at the business of de-tangling and therefore aiding the business of removing nits and lice back at the *gîte*.

But should you opt for the chemical route, who is brave enough to face those stern pharmacists in their spike-heeled court shoes and lab coats in the pristine *pharmacies* where narry a furry hot water bottle cover nor novelty baby bib can be found? Unlike in the UK, I think those independent chemists survive because *les supermarchés* are too scared of them to stock more than two bottles of conditioner. And once the product is secured, do you understand the instructions? *Non*.

Have comb, will travel. I have combed in restrooms, on boats, in courtyards and on beaches and I have to admit, nothing beats the thrill of finding neither nits nor lice on holiday.

Lousy Help When Abroad: Foreign Vocabulary

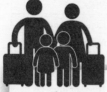

Oi, Stop scratching!	Hé, arrête de gratter!
I'm feeling lousy today.	Je ne suis pas en forme aujourd'hui.
Our head lice are more insecticide-resistant than yours.	Notre poux de tête sont plus résistants aux insecticides que les vôtres.
Waiter, there is a head louse in my soup.	Garçon, il y a un pou de tête dans ma soupe.
Can you direct me to the nearest pub?	Ou se trouve la pub la plus proche?
I shake hands so I can't get head lice from you foreign chappies.	Je te serre la main pour ne pas attraper tes poux de tête.
The English are always scratching their heads.	Les Anglais se creusent toujours la tête.

Vocabulary		
English	*French*	**German**
nit (louse egg)	*lente*	**Nisse**
head louse/lice	*pou/poux de tête*	**Kopflaus/Läuse**
nit comb	*peigne à poux/ peigne anti poux*	**Nissenkamm**
fine-toothed comb	*peigne fin*	**feiner Kamm**
hair conditioner	*démêlant*	**Haarspülung**
shampoo	*shampooing*	**Shampoo**
to scratch	*gratter*	**Kratzen**
to itch	*démanger*	**Juckreiz**

Phrases: 1) English, 2) *French*, 3) German

1) I'd like to buy a nit comb please.
2) *Je voudrais acheter un peigne anti poux s'il vous plaît.*
3) Ich möchte bitte einem Nissenkamm kaufen.

1) Do you have anything to treat head lice?
2) *Avez-vous un traitement pour les poux de tête?*
3) Haben Sie etwas gegen Kopfläuse?

1) I found several adult lice.
2) *J'ai trouvé plusieurs poux adultes.*
3) Ich habe einige ausgewachsene Läuse gefunden.

1) Nits are just the empty egg shells.
2) *Les lentes sont des coquilles d'œufs vides.*
3) Nissen sind einfach die leeren Eierschalen.

1) It is the live lice you need to look for.
2) *C'est les poux vivants que vous devez chercher.*
3) Sie müssen die lebende Läuse suchen.

1) No that is just a silly myth.
2) *Non, ceci n'est qu'un mythe bête.*
3) Doch, das ist ein dummer Mythos.

1) I've read *The Little Book of Nits* and I know what I'm talking about.
2) *J'ai lu Le Petit Livre des Poux, et je sais de quoi je parle.*
3) Ich habe das *Kleine Buch der Läuse* gelesen, und ich weiß, wovon ich rede.

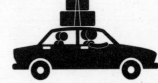

Lice in Art and Literature

THE LICE SEEKERS

When the child's forehead, full of torments red
Implores the swarm of white dreams hovering dim,
Two elder sisters take him from his bed,
Sisters with silvery nails and slim,

He hears their black lids beating; and their mild,
Electric fingers, in the scented breath
Of silence that in greyness folds the child,
On royal nails crack little lice to death.

by Arthur Rimbaud (1851–1891)
translated by Jethro Bithell (d.1938), 1912

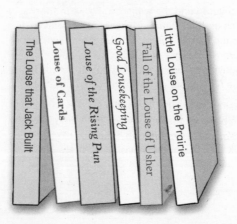

The Louse that Jack Built

Louse of Cards

Louse of the Rising Pun

Good Lousekeeping

Fall of the Louse of Usher

Little Louse on the Prairie

Throughout history, artists have sought to depict lice in some way, whether through the medium of prose such as our French friend opposite, or visually. *The Garden of Health*, published in 1491, shows a man on his knees being brushed by a lady while three over-sized lice run around a water bowl.

In India, a temple finished in 1546 has a panel showing a husband lying on a bed as his wife plucks lice from his hair. In Tintoretto's *Susanna and the Elders* from the mid-16th century, we find an ornate two-sided comb and Caravaggio also included a double-sided comb in *Martha and Mary Magdalene* (*c.* 1596). The Dutch school was especially keen to reflect the realities of everyday life and several famous paintings show subjects delousing each other.

Christopher Marlow, a contemporary of Shakespeare, refers to lice and stavesacre in his drama, *Doctor Faustus*. In 1728, Jonathan Swift wrote:

> *When you saw Tady at long bullets play,*
> *You sate and loused him all a sunshine day:*
> *How could you, Sheelah, listen to his tales,*
> *Or crack such lice as his between your nails?*

These days, children find the subject fun to read thanks to writers such as John Dougherty who has a head louse called Jim as the hero in *Niteracy Hour*, Francesca Simon who added *Horrid Henry's Nits* to her series about the infamous eponymous rascal, and Australian author Tristan Bancks whose *Nit Boy* series has also been animated.

In the summer of 2011, *The Itch of the Golden Nit*, a collaboration between the Tate, Aardman Animations (the creators of *Wallace & Gromit*) and hundreds of children across the UK was shown on television.

To a Louse

Ha! whaur ye gaun, ye crowlin ferlie?
Your impudence protects you sairly;
I canna say but ye strunt rarely,
Owre gauze and lace;
Tho', faith! I fear ye dine but sparely
On sic a place.

Ye ugly, creepin, blastit wonner,
Detested, shunn'd by saunt an' sinner,
How daur ye set your fit upon her –
Sae fine a lady?
Gae somewhere else and seek your dinner
On some poor body.

Swith! in some beggar's haffet squattle;
There ye may creep, and sprawl, and sprattle,
Wi' ither kindred, jumping cattle,
In shoals and nations;
Whaur horn nor bane ne'er daur unsettle
Your thick plantations.

Now haud you there, ye're out o' sight,
Below the fatt'rels, snug and tight;
Na, faith ye yet! ye'll no be right,
Till ye've got on it –
The verra tapmost, tow'rin height
O' Miss' bonnet.
My sooth! right bauld ye set your nose out,

*Inspired by seeing a louse crawling on the bonnet of a lady sitting in front of him in church, Burns is likely to have been describing a body louse on the move, rather than a head louse.

As plump an' grey as ony groset:
O for some rank, mercurial rozet,
Or fell, red smeddum,
I'd gie you sic a hearty dose o't,
Wad dress your droddum.

I wad na been surpris'd to spy
You on an auld wife's flainen toy;
Or aiblins some bit dubbie boy,
On's wyliecoat;
But Miss' fine Lunardi! fye!
How daur ye do't?

O Jeany, dinna toss your head,
An' set your beauties a' abread!
Ye little ken what cursed speed
The blastie's makin:
Thae winks an' finger-ends, I dread,
Are notice takin.

O wad some Power the giftie gie us
To see oursels as ithers see us!
It wad frae mony a blunder free us,
An' foolish notion:
What airs in dress an' gait wad lea'e us,
An' ev'n devotion!

by Robert Burns (1785)*

'Love this poem … had to recite it, aged 10, in front of the whole primary school. Ah, memories. To be honest, we weren't really sure what it was about, as we called them nits. Think it took a few years to dawn on me that I'd been reciting a poem about head lice!'

Sarah Litchfield, herself now a primary school teacher

VAMPIRE BUGS

Head lice suck blood. Quite a lot of other insects like our blood, too. There are fleas, bed-bugs, mosquitoes, midges, and a small brown moth called *Calyptra eustrigata*. Not to mention the non-insect groups like ticks, chiggers (skin-burrowing mites) and leaches.

Blood is good food. It is high in protein, with all those red blood corpuscles full of haemoglobin, and the serum fluid filled with complex biochemicals. And as it's a watery liquid, it is easily sucked up without any need to bite or chew.

But contrary to ideas put about in romantic teen vampire fiction, blood is not the perfect diet and eating blood alone will lead to nutritional deficiencies. Blood-feeders like mosquitoes eat blood only as adults. As larvae, they get a whole other set of nutrients from the decaying organic matter on which they feed. Blood is just a top-up food to mature their eggs. But head lice feed on blood alone and they need extra help. They get this from micro-organisms living inside their bodies.

The head louse has special pockets called mycetomes attached to its guts. These are full of dedicated bacteria. They digest the blood differently and supply the louse with vitamins and other chemicals it cannot produce on its own. Depriving a louse of its live-in bacteria severely limits its growth, and may kill it. Surely there's a louse-remedy research project there somewhere?

Not all blood is equally acceptable to a louse, though. Alligator blood cells are too big to pass up the louse's snout, for example. Guinea pig haemoglobin crystallises in the gut and rips the louse intestines open. Human blood, though, is just right∗

BLOOD LOSS

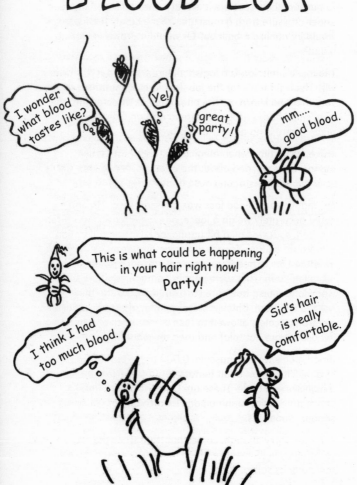

Critters by Ivydale Primary School, Natural History Club.

Y**OU** have to respect an animal that bites something 100 million times larger than itself. But you also have to question how sensible it is to try and tap blood pumped under pressure from a muscular heart. Surely the louse would inflate like a balloon? Or would it drown in leaking blood?

The louse's mission is a logistical nightmare, but it is armed with the right tools for the job. Its piercing mouthparts are very thin and sharp. As the biting tube is inserted into the skin, small hooks around it extend and anchor the louse in place. There is no danger of a blow-out.

There was a time when medical textbooks and louse monographs worried about the effects of blood loss. Could severe louse infestation cause anaemia?

For many years, blood loss was guesstimated. No one could accurately weigh a louse, or even discover how often they fed, so it was all a bit haphazard. Finally, Australian phthirapterist Rick Speare did some proper measurements in 2006. Lots of head lice were collected from helpful schoolchildren. They were kept in humane conditions, warm and moist, but were starved for six hours (the lice, not the children). Batches were weighed on super-accurate electronic scales, allowed to feed on the back of a hand (whose we are not told) and then reweighed.

Blood meals were minuscule: 0.0001579 (that's $1/6000$) of a millilitre in an adult female, 0.0000657 ($1/15,000$) of a millilitre in a male. These are truly trivial amounts. Thousands of lice biting all day long could not cause serious blood loss.

The real worry, though, comes not from what the louse takes away in its meagre blood meal, but what it leaves behind in its saliva.

CLOG-FREE DRINKING

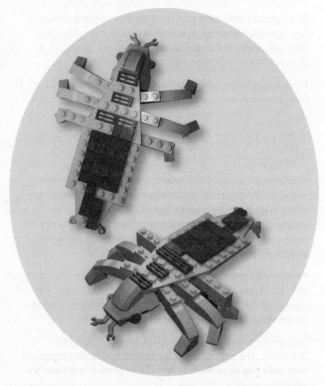

If you make a Lego head louse, remember to use some red bricks to show its blood-filled intestines snaking through its translucent body.

Human blood clots easily. Otherwise, even the slightest nick shaving or chopping the vegetables would put us in mortal danger as it all leaked away. A complex biochemical reactions starts in a fraction of a second if even the tiniest capillary blood vessel is damaged. Even if it is bitten into by a head louse. By all reports, the louse should just get a mouthful of wet scab. But the louse is ahead of the game, and instead drinks its fill.

To stop our blood clogging up their fine sucking mouthparts, head lice wage chemical war on us. As they suck, they also inject saliva full of anticoagulants to stop the blood cells clotting together. It works perfectly.

In seriously heavy infestations (that's many hundreds of lice), a person may be receiving thousands of bites each day. The human immune system eventually starts reacting to all the injected louse saliva. The victim has a slightly raised temperature, they feel achy, lethargic, irritable and genuinely unwell; they feel, in a word, *lousy*.

Children suffering in this way become tired, sullen and withdrawn. They can't concentrate and in less enlightened times were branded *nitwits* by their teachers. It was thought that head lice preferred less intelligent heads, but it now turns out that louse saliva was interfering with the children's education.

All that biting on the head – and the scratching that goes with it – takes a toll on the skin, too. It makes the scalp feel tight and dull, feeling and sensation are reduced and the victim is becoming, quite literally, a *numbskull*.

Louse researchers still have to be careful of allergic reactions. The dry, dusty louse faeces can cause coughing and sneezing (just like hay fever) if too much gets into the laboratory air.

Head lice only on Heads? Yes.

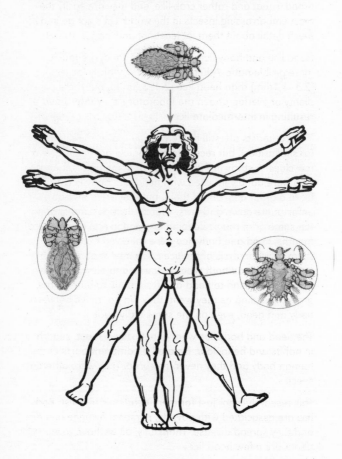

Humans are home to three louse species: head lice, body lice and crab lice (also called pubic lice). Each has its own favoured blood-sucking spot on the delicate human body.

Crab lice are easy to differentiate. They are small (1.1–1.9mm), broad, squat and rather crab-like, and they are easily the most embarrassing insects in the world. Let's not go into too much detail about them, at least not until pages 108–9.

Head lice and body lice, on the other hand, are much more problematic. Adult body lice are slightly larger (2.3–4.1mm) than head lice (2.1–3.3mm), but there is plenty of overlap and in the laboratory, they interbreed resulting in intermediate lice.

Phthirapterists are still politely arguing over the differences (or similarities), but recent technological advances give a few clues. A study in 2005 looked at some unfortunates who were doubly infested with head and body lice. We don't learn a great deal about them, but they were probably unfortunate down-and-outs, wretchedly poor and sharing the same grim rough-sleeping arrangements. Over several months, head and body lice were collected from each of them. DNA analysis of the lice confirmed that although each person had both types of louse, and although they moved from head to head and from body to body in the group, breeding as they went, they did not move between body and head, even on the same individual.

The head and body lice were genetically distinct, separate in habits and behaviour, isolated on different parts of the human body and they never interbred. They were different species.

This research is not just for mere academic interest. Body lice are associated with poverty, personal hygiene and dirt, and they spread disease. Thankfully, all we have to worry about are a few head lice

BODY LICE?
JUST TAKE OFF
YOUR CLOTHES

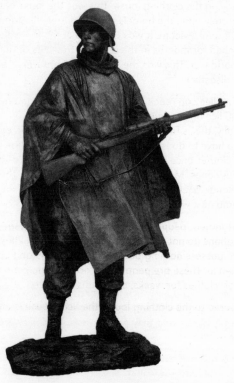

The body louse is the louse of war, famine and homelessness,
the louse of the natural and the man-made disaster.

The body louse would be better called the *clothing louse*. One of its older scientific names, *Pediculus vestimenti*, echoes this. Most of the time, clothing lice hide in the dense weave of the clothes but move to the skin to feed four or five times a day. Just like head lice, they carefully glue their nits in place, but they attach them to the clothing fibres rather than to body hairs.

Much of what we know about lice today was discovered by studying the clothing louse. This was the louse of the desperately poor, the homeless, the refugee, the famine or earthquake victim. It was the louse of the foot soldier encamped for months in the cold wet trenches during the first world war. This was the louse of the natural or man-made disaster.

Clothing lice can reach appalling proportions and finding 30,000 lice on a single person was all too common. Yet ironically, this is the louse that is easiest to get rid of. All you have to do is take off your clothes. A change into clean clothes once a week will allow you to wash and air the lousy ones. Most lice and nits will be dead by the time you change back. Or if they are not, the few survivors will succumb next week.

Unfortunately, people suffering from clothing-louse infestations do not own a second set of clothes. They may, in fact, possess nothing but the clothes they stand up in, or lie down in. These are people who do not, who *cannot*, take off their clothes for weeks, or months or years.

Compared to the clothing louse, the head louse is a doddle.

BODY LICE?
NO, THANKS!

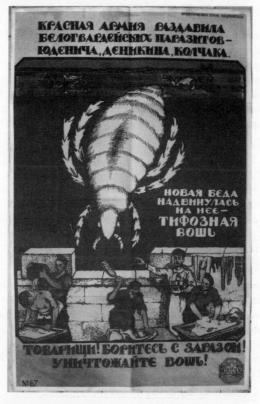

Russian anti-louse poster, text reads: 'Red Army squashed
White Army's parasites: Yudenich,Denikin, Kolchak. Now
the Red Army has a new trouble – typhus louse! Comrades,
fight with this infection! Do away with the louse!'

With the exception of malaria mosquitoes, the clothing or body louse has killed more people than any other animal on the planet. It has killed them by spreading three important diseases.

Typhus[*] (*Rickettsia prowazekii*) is a bacterium causing fever, aches, cough, weakness and a blotchy rash. Some 'plagues' of the Middle Ages are likely to have been typhus, spread by lice, rather than the bubonic disease spread by fleas. A body louse drinking blood from a diseased person becomes infected as the microbes breed in its guts. The bacteria damage the insect's intestines and the louse starts to pass copious bloody bacterial faeces. If the diseased louse moves on to another person, the faeces infect small cuts in the skin, which are usually the result of scratching. Depending on the strain of bacteria up to 60% of human victims die unless treated with antibiotics. Head lice, though, do not carry disease.

Trench fever (*Bartonella quintana*) is a similar organism, spread by body lice in a similar way. It is not usually fatal but is still unpleasant and debilitating. It came to prominence in the infantry soldiers huddled in the trenches of the first world war. Head lice, though, do not carry disease.

Relapsing fever (*Borrelia recurrentis*) is another type of bacterium. This time, the bacteria reproduce and lodge inside the louse's body. They are released only if the body louse is crushed at the site of the itchy bites – a common enough event. Human mortality can reach 10% unless this disease is treated with antibiotics. Head lice, though, do not carry disease.

One more time. *Head lice do not carry disease.*

---

[*]Not to be confused with *typhoid*, another bacterium *Salmonella typhii*, spread in contaminated food or water.

Don't Mention
Crabs

No use standing on the seat Brighton* crabs can jump 10 feet.

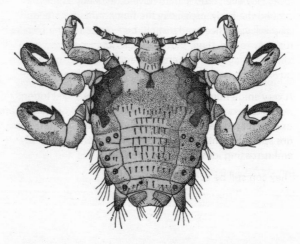

*You can substitute the name of any town you like here – crabs aren't fussy.

Crab lice are so named for obvious reasons. They are broad, fat, stout lice and with extra-large heavy claws on their middle and back legs, there is definitely something crab-like about them. They are also called the pubic louse for other obvious reasons: they inhabit the nether regions. Here, they cause intense itching and the bites can become inflamed, causing small raised purple spots. Needless to say, crabs are also the most embarrassing lice, and rarely talked of in polite society.

It's not really that crab lice have a predilection for the groin and their spread by casual sex is sometimes over-emphasised. It is more to do with the fact that they have broader bodies and stouter claws, adapted for clinging to the coarse, more widely-spaced pubic hairs rather than the finer and closer scalp hairs.

Just like head and body lice, they get around by physical contact, in this case usually in shared double beds. The French called them *papillons d'amour* ➤ 'butterflies of love'. However, crab lice do have a tendency to wander around the body, especially the hairy human male, and they will visit chest and armpit, beard and moustache. It's easy to see, then, that they can get transferred onto innocent victims and there are regular reports of children having crab louse infestations in the eyelashes.

A very small number (less than 1%) of louse infestations on heads turn out to be crab lice. These unusual outbreaks are usually on red-headed people, whose thicker hair strands are spaced slightly further apart. This is an exceedingly embarrassing louse.

They can still be combed out though.

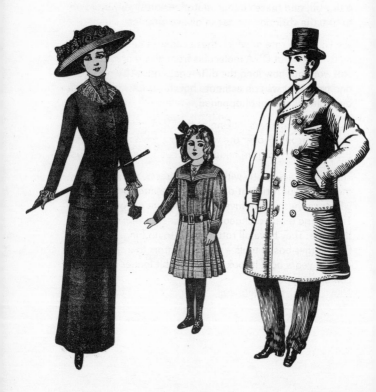

When Did We Start Wearing Clothes?

S tudying head lice can tell us some remarkable things about our own history ⟶ such as when humans first started wearing clothes. There was always an assumption that body lice evolved from head lice in response to the 'new' human fashion of wearing clothes, rather than walking around naked. Now we have firm evidence not just that this occurred, but *when* it occurred.

DNA, the stuff of our genes, can now be examined at the molecular level. This is the DNA sequencing often used in evidence in court cases, or at least in TV dramas. The molecules of DNA sometimes get damaged or altered, just a tiny bit, and these chance mutations gradually build up to give the variation we see in all living things.

We know the rate at which these changes occur naturally. So by looking at DNA molecules from different animals, we can work out how long the differences have taken to occur, and from that we can estimate how far backwards in time an evolutionary split happened.

In 2003, researchers looking at the DNA of head lice and body lice from all over the world made a clear discovery. Body lice evolved from head lice about 72,000 years ago.

This fits in very neatly with the fact that humans started moving out of Africa at about this time into cooler regions where clothes would have been a definite advantage. There is no direct archaeological evidence of clothes from this time. They have all rotted away to nothing. But the first clothes-based tools – needles – start to appear about 40,000 years ago. It took just a little bit longer for nit combs to appear.

Keeping Lice *as* Pets

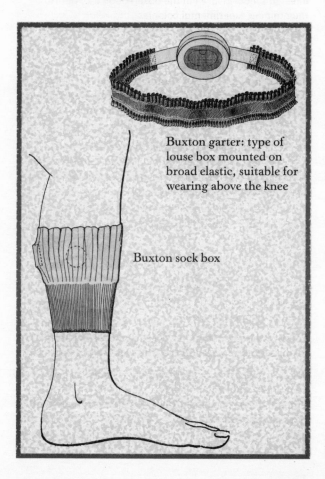

Buxton garter: type of louse box mounted on broad elastic, suitable for wearing above the knee

Buxton sock box

We know quite a lot about louse lives — the different sex ratios, preferences for temperature and humidity, daily and nightly movements, feeding rates, sexual foreplay, egg-hatching and survival rates. We know this not from randomly checking lousy heads or keeping infested schoolchildren in the observation lab, but from maintaining experimental colonies.

Louse researchers have tirelessly dedicated their own bodies to the advancement of science and have kept the insects they study as personal pets. It is possible to keep lice in a glass tube with a twist of damp paper, but they have to be kept warm and they have to be let out onto the skin to feed at least twice a day. It's all a bit fiddly and not ideal. It's better to *wear* the lice.

Delicately crafted cardboard boxes in which to house lice were first made by bacteriologist George Nuttall and described to an eager louse research world in 1917. The bottom of the box was cut out and lined with fine silk with a tight, regular mesh. It was developed for milling flour but proved perfect for keeping the lice in whilst allowing them to feed through it.

Several boxes of lice could be worn in the sock-top, although, as was pointed out, this is hardly compatible with a short skirt and silk stockings. Female researchers were not let off, though, and a stylish louse garter was created to be worn above the knee.

Polish phthirapterist Rudolf Weigl employed 50 people to feed his stock of 350,000 lice. This was big business.

Today, it is possible to keep laboratory head lice in enclosed containers and let them feed on stored human blood through an artificial membrane. It's all a bit impersonal and antiseptic though.

The Fascination of Lice

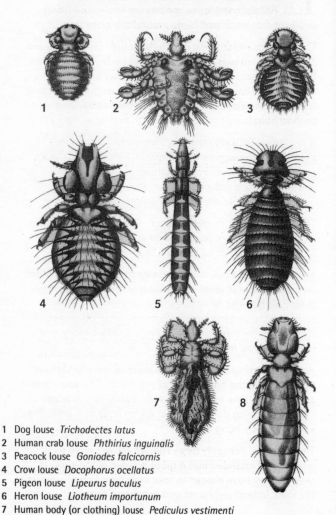

1 Dog louse *Trichodectes latus*
2 Human crab louse *Phthirius inguinalis*
3 Peacock louse *Goniodes falcicornis*
4 Crow louse *Docophorus ocellatus*
5 Pigeon louse *Lipeurus baculus*
6 Heron louse *Liotheum importunum*
7 Human body (or clothing) louse *Pediculus vestimenti*
8 Swan louse *Ornithobius cygnorum*

Lice are fascinating, ask any phthirapterist. Over 3,200 different louse species are known, infesting different mammals and birds around the globe.

Chewing lice infest birds, mostly, although some are found on cats, guinea-pigs, cattle, goats, horses and sheep. They have large, broad heads and chewing jaws with which to scrape skin. They usually have two claws at the end of each leg rather than one: maybe feathers need more clinging on to than hairs?

It is a marvellous mystery why *Harrisoniella irroratae*, the louse of the wandering albatross, has only four legs rather than the usual insect number of six. What should be its front pair are reduced to short stumps and instead it 'walks' by using its over-large antennae.

The pelican louse, *Piagetiella titan*, lives inside the bird's peculiar beak. Every so often, however, it returns to the bird's head to lay its eggs in the feathers.

Sucking lice have pointed blood-sucking mouthparts. Most mammals have at least one species of louse feeding on them. We humans have three. The exceptions are the carnivores, apart from the unfortunate dog, otter, seals, walrus and (by an odd quirk of evolutionary history and plate tectonics) marsupials.

Antarctophthirus ogmorhini, the louse of the Weddell seal has, perhaps, the hardest life of any insect. The seals spend most of their time in Antarctic seas, swimming in water at −2°C, and diving down to 450m for an hour at a time. The lice can barely hang on.

The 'snouted' lice (only three species known) have their entire head extended into a giant pointed blood-sucking skewer. They have chosen to take their blood meals through the thick hide of elephants and warthogs. Respect!

The Little Book of Louse Records

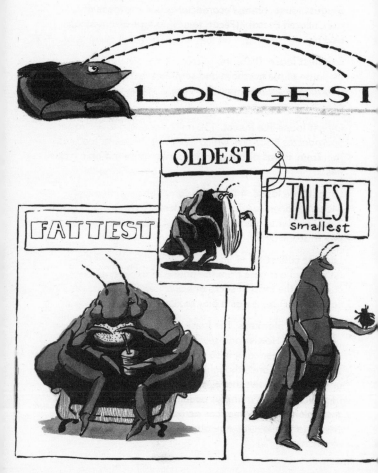

Largest infestation. You might think one head louse is too many. Spare a thought for the schoolchild discovered by Australian phthirapterist Rick Speare, who had 2,657 lice in his or her hair. This is a record ➔ unless you know different.

Biggest louse. 8mm, *Pecaroecus javalii*, the louse of the Collared Peccary (Pecari tajacu), a type of American wild pig.

Smallest louse. 0.35mm, *Microphthirus uncinatus*, the louse of the northern and southern flying squirrels (*Glaucomys sabrinus* and *G. volans*) in North and Central America.

Oldest louse-like insect. 130-million-year-old fossil named *Saurodectes vrsanskyi*, which has some louse-like features. At 17mm, it was also a giant and must have fed on a giant host.

Oldest true louse. 44-million-year-old fossil called *Megamenopon rasnitsyni*. The oldest known genuine louse, similar to modern feather lice, it probably fed on a prehistoric bird.

Largest collection of lice. It is said that the Aztec rulers demanded a tribute from the poorest members of their society in the form of sacks of head lice. There was no value in the lice; it was a ploy to keep idle fingers busy.

Unluckiest monkeys. The louse *Pediculus mjöbergi* occurs on Capucin, Howler and several other monkeys in Central and South America. It is so similar to human head lice that they were once thought to be the same species. DNA analysis now shows that *P. mjobergi* evolved from human head lice and the monkeys acquired them from the humans that colonised the Americas across the Bering Strait from Asia after the last Ice Age about 15,000 years ago. Poor old monkeys.

Knitted Nits

You need:
4mm (size 8) knitting needles
A scrap of double-knit wool (*c.* 2m) in pink or red

Abbreviations:
inc – increase
k2tog – knit two stitches together

loop – to make a loop, start knitting into the next stitch on the left-hand needle, i.e. insert the right-hand needle into the stitch, bring the yarn over the needle and pull it through, so that there's a new stitch on the right hand needle. Now, instead of sliding the stitch off the left-hand needle, bring the yarn forward between the needles, wrap it twice around your left thumb to create a loop (aim for a loop about 4cm long) and, holding your loop in place, take the yarn back between the needles. Knit into the stitch which remains on the left hand needle and slide it off, as usual. You've now made two stitches on the right-hand needle; to fix the loop, bring the first (right hand) stitch over the second (left hand) stitch, as if you were casting off. Give the loop a tug to tighten it, then carry on knitting.

Cast on 3 stitches, leaving a long tail.

Row 1: k1, inc, k1 (4 stitches)
Row 2: k1, inc, inc, k1 (6 stitches)
Row 3: k6
Row 4: k1, inc, k2, inc, k1 (8 stitches)
Row 5: k8
Row 6: k1, inc, k4, inc, k1 (10 stitches)

Row 7:   k10
Row 8:   k2, make a loop into 3rd stitch, k4, make a loop
              into 8th stitch, k2
Row 9:   k10
Row 10: k2, loop, k4, loop, k2
Row 11: (k2tog) x 5 (5 stitches)
Row 12: k1, loop, k1, loop, k1
Row 13: k2tog, k1, k2tog (3 stitches)
Row 14: k3
Row 15: k3tog (1 stitch)

Draw the yarn through the remaining stitch, pull tight and cut off, sewing the end in.

Use the long tail to sew up the central seam of the nit, matching the two sides up and joining them together (make sure that the legs are on the outside). When you're half way up, stuff the body lightly (you can use a left-over bit of wool for this), then sew up to the top and finish off. Clip the yarn short, leaving a 3mm end to make a 'mouth' for your nit.

Finally, tie a knot in each of the legs and clip the ends off, so that they're all the same length.

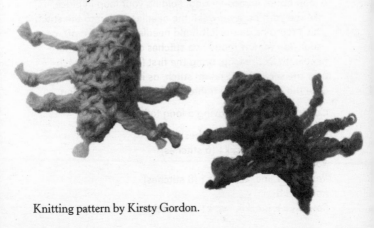

Knitting pattern by Kirsty Gordon.

A FEW FINAL WORDS...

Japanese haiku

Fleas, lice
A horse peeing
Near my pillow

by Matsuo Basho (1644–1695)

So there you have it. Head lice can be annoying but they can be defeated. And like most enemies, they are best defeated by first understanding them.

Armed with the information in this book, we hope that you'll now be better equipped for the louse hunts ahead.

Look – First, look for your head lice. Know what they look like, how big they are and where they live. Don't fuss about nits: it's the *live head lice* you need to be worried about.

Find – Don't be alarmed if you find head lice. Children get them all the time. So do parents. So do teachers. Once found, they can be got rid of.

Remove – Repeated combing is the secret to success. Use a specially designed nit comb. Concentrate on the scalp and comb through *and out* to remove them.

Use whatever works for you and your children – dry hair, wet hair, conditioner, hair oil, short-toothed comb, long-toothed comb, you name it. The main thing is that you get the action right and the time to do it thoroughly without fighting a reluctant child. If you must use a chemical treatment, make sure it is one that works and that it is an insecticide recommended by doctors. None of those currently available is claimed to be 100% effective, so combine whatever you use with combing. Repeat as necessary. Repeat.

Rejoice – Hooray. You will have a louse-free house ... until the next time. Keep vigilant, look regularly, comb regularly. Don't fret. Don't panic.

Eat Only If Really Necessary

Warning – do not eat your lice, unless you are a monkey.

What would happen in a world without nits? Well, you wouldn't be reading this book for a start! We hope you found *The Little Book of Nits* entertaining and helpful.

Good hunting!

Louse Lexicon

Louse Any small, mean, annoying critter, but more especially the *head louse* ⟵ a wingless, blood-sucking insect that frequently inhabits the scalps of children (and sometimes adults), where it causes itching and scratching. It can also raise the blood-pressure of frustrated parents, leading to outbursts of bad temper and swearing. Plural *lice*, as in rhymes with 'not very nice'.

Louse-ladders Jackspeak (naval slang) for sideburns.

Lousy Infested with lice. Also *feeling lousy*, being irritable, listless and sullen, often accompanied by slightly raised temperature and flu-like aches, caused by the body's immune response to multiple doses of louse saliva injected as an anticoagulant to prevent blood-clots during louse feeding.

Nit Insect egg, more specifically the egg of the head louse super-glued to a hair strand. Even more specifically, the *empty* egg shell which lingers longer than expected, causing unnecessary anxiety to school boards.

Nit-picker Mother (occasionally a father or older sibling) who grooms head lice from young ones. Also *nit-picking*, the act of careful, precise, patient and tolerant grooming.

Nitty-gritty Dust-dry louse faeces, often disturbed by the head-scratching louse-infested pupil struggling over reading, 'riting and 'rithmetic.

Nit-wit A dolt. Someone whose wits are dimmed by chronic allergic reaction to louse bites. Originally a simpleton whose low intelligence obviously attracted more head lice. Not to be confused with *knit-wit*, someone who tells jokes about knitting.

Nitty Nora The nit nurse. However, there are grave doubts that one was ever called Nora. There are also doubts that there were ever specific 'nit' nurses, just that school nurses' other tasks have not been so immortalised.

No-nits policy Ill-advised guidelines for excluding from school children with empty louse eggs in their hair. Much easier to enforce than a no-living-lice policy.

Numbskull A nit-wit, one whose scalp has become desensitised, tight and numb in response to continued multiple louse bites during heavy infestations.

Phthiraptera Official, scientific name for the insect group which includes human head lice, and also the weird and wonderful lice of many other mammals and birds.

Phthirapterist Cool-sounding job title of a scientist who studies lice. A nit-picker.

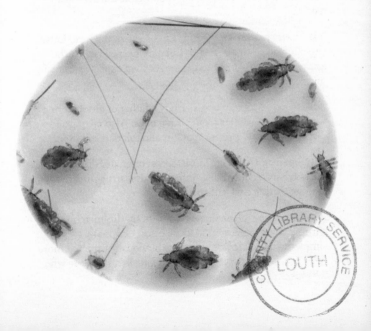

Lice Fanatics:
Websites and Reads

Books and pamphlets

Adamson, J. 2011. *Topsy & Tim Have Itchy Heads*. London: Ladybird.

Bancks, Tristan. 2009. *Bug Out*. Mosman, New South Wales: Laguna Bay Books.

Bancks, Tristan. 2009. *Lift Off*. Mosman, New South Wales: Laguna Bay Books.

Buxton, P.A. 1939. *The Louse: An Account of the Lice Which Infest Man, Their Medical Importance and Control*. London: Edward Arnold & Co. Reprinted 1947. Long out of print, but second-hand or print-to-order copies are available.

Denny, H. 1842. *Monographia Anoplurum Britanniae: Or, an Essay on the British Species of Parasitic Insects Belonging to the Order Anoplura of Leach... etc*. London: Henry G. Bohn. Rare, even in specialist antiquarian bookshops, but the first major work on lice in English.

Dougherty, J. 2005. *Niteracy Hour*. London: Young Corgi.

Ferris, G. F. 1951. *The Sucking Lice*. San Francisco: Memoirs of the Pacific Coast Entomological Society, Volume 1.

Kim, K.C., Pratt, H.D. & Stojanovich, C.J. 1986. *The Sucking Lice of North America: An Illustrated Manual for Identification*. State College, PA: Penn State University Press.

Simon, F. 1997. *Horrid Henry's Nits*. Orion Children's Books.

Smart, J. 1942. *Lice*. London: Trustees of the British Museum. First written at time of war, this pamphlet was reprinted in 1948 and 1954.

Articles

Burgess, I.F. 2004. Human Lice and their Control. *Annual Review of Entomology* 49: 457–581.

Maunder, J.W. 1983. The Appreciation of Lice. *Proceedings of the Royal Institution of Great Britain* 55: 1–31.

Websites

Nit Heads – *The Wonderful World of Head Lice*:
www.lousehead.wordpress.com
Richard & Justine's very own lousy blog

Phthiraptera.info:
www.phthiraptera.info
The website of the International Society of Phthirapterists
(for louse specialists this one)

Tree of life – Phthiraptera:
www.tolweb.org/phthiraptera/8237
Collaborative collection of web pages examining animal
biodiversity

NHS direct:
http://www.nhs.uk/Conditions/Head-lice/Pages/
Introduction.aspx
Standard UK health advice and information on head lice.

Acknowledgements

Finally, we'd like to thank: Rebecca Palmer (www.bepalmer. blogspot.com) for the excellent cartoons on pages 20, 28, 44, 58, 64 and 82; Sadie Hennessy (www.sadiehennessy.co.uk) for the nit magnet postcard on page 32; Kirsty Gordon for the nit knitting pattern on page 118 and the children of Ivydale Primary School, Natural History Club, for the drawings on page 98, and Franck Cassedanne and Lukas Schwimann, who advised on the translations on pages 90–1.

Artwork

Contents, ElenaMaria/Shutterstock; 9, Robert Hooke/ Wiki Media; 10, Susan McIntyre; 19, Francesco Abrignani/ Shutterstock; 20, Rebecca Palmer; 22, head louse–3drenderings/ Shutterstock; 28, Rebecca Palmer; 32, Sadie Hennessy; 38, head louse–3drenderings/Shutterstock; 40, head louse–3drenderings/ Shutterstock; 42, lian_2011/Shutterstock; 44, Rebecca Palmer; 50, Glenn Kershner/Shutterstock; 57, Morphart/Shutterstock; 58, Rebecca Palmer; 64, Rebecca Palmer; 68, head louse– 3drenderings/Shutterstock; 70, Accent/Shutterstock; 74–75, comb–Susan McIntyre; 76, dmiskv/Shutterstock; 82, Rebecca Palmer; 86, advent/Shutterstock; 90–91 Leremy/Shutterstock; 92, Susan McIntyre; 98, Ivydale Primary School; 102, Thank You/ Shutterstock; 110 left and middle, AKaiser/Shutterstock; 110 right, jumpingsack/Shutterstock; 116, Rebecca Palmer.

Photographs

11, Mauro Rodrigues/Shutterstock; 12, Eye of Science/Science Photo Library; 22, nymph–KevinDyer/iStockphoto; 22, nit comb–Richard Jones and Justine Crow; 24, marekuliasz/ Shutterstock; 30, Gary Hunter/Wellcome Images; 38, Tristan3D/ Shutterstock; 40, Costas/Shutterstock; 48, RetroClipArt/ Shutterstock; 52, Richard Jones and Justine Crow; 60, Africa Studio/Shutterstock; 61, Margrit Hirsch/Shutterstock; 62, Lukiyanova Natalia / frenta/Shutterstock; 72, Richard Jones and Justine Crow; 80, KevinDyer/iStockphoto; 100, Richard Jones and Justine Crow; 104, rorem/Shutterstock; 119, Richard Jones and Justine Crow; 123, KevinDyer/iStockphoto.

Index